MW01223785

MY RADHA BEAUTY

Essential Oils

Aromatherapy Diffuser Handbook

★

200 Recipes and Everything You Need to Get Started With Aromatherapy Cool Mist Diffusion for Mind, Body, and Spirit

by Cassandra Kiernan

My Radha Beauty Essential Oils Aromatherapy Diffuser Handbook:
200 Recipes and Everything You Need to Get Started With
Aromatherapy Cool Mist Diffusion for Mind, Body, and Spirit

Copyright © 2016 Cassandra Kiernan

Cover photo credit:
peshkova/ Depositphotos.com

Book design by Velin@Perseus-Design.com

Back cover: mimagephotos/ Depositphotos.com

All rights reserved.

The use of any part of this publication reproduced, transmitted
in any form or by any means, electronic, mechanical, recording
or otherwise, or stored in a retrieval system, without the prior
consent of the publisher is an infringement of the copyright
law. In the case of photocopying or other reprographic copying of
the material, a license must be obtained before proceeding.

Radha Beauty is the registered trademark of Radha Beauty Products LLC.
Radha Beauty offers the best products and the best customer service.

Legal Disclaimer

The information contained in this book is the opinion of the author
and is based on the author's personal experience and observations.
The author does not assume liability whatsoever for the use of or
inability to use any or all information contained in this book, and
accepts no responsibility for any loss or damages of any kind that may
be incurred by the reader as a result of actions arising from the use
of information in this book. Use this information at your own risk.
The author reserves the right to make any changes he or she deems
necessary to future versions of the publication to ensure its accuracy.

CONTENTS

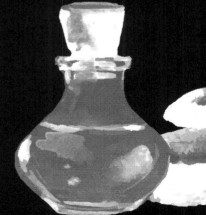

BODY 61

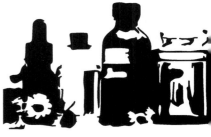

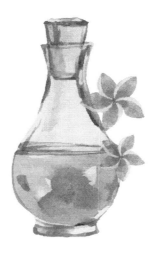

SPIRIT 141

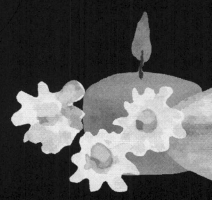

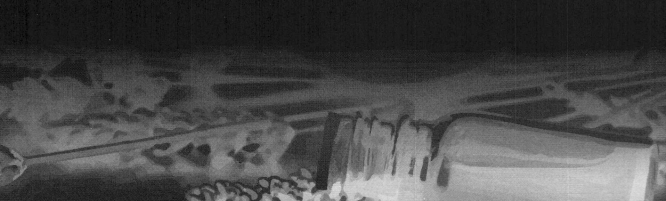

INTRODUCTION

Of all our five senses developed over millennia of human existence, the sense of smell is the oldest and most primal. Our mental, physical, and spiritual connections to the fragrances and aromas in nature are inextricably linked to our survival and well being.

It's a strange fallacy to think of aromatherapy as a "new age" practice. In actual fact, the use of fragrances to heal and treat the human condition forms the basis of all medicine as we know it. As far back as the days of the pharaohs in ancient Egypt, and the empire of Huang Ti in China, essential oils have been extracted from certain plants for their powerful properties. Hippocrates, the ancient Greek father of modern medicine, was also the first known holistic healer, treating the entire body as a whole organism, and documenting uses for more than 200 natural compounds.

This book combines that ancient wisdom with personal knowledge built on decades of experience in aromatherapy, to present 200 essential oil recipes to treat the mind, body, and spirit. While none of these blends can be treated as medical advice or prescriptions, they offer powerful and effective guidelines for living a happier, healthier, and more enlightened life.

Mother Nature has given us all necessary gifts to thrive in this world – and then some. All we have to do is put it together. This book is your manual for doing so.

HOW TO USE THIS BOOK

These pages are written as a practical reference for aromatherapy beginners and experts alike. The recipes are organized loosely in order of their applications ("Mind", "Body", "Spirit"), so that you can easily access exactly what you're looking for.

Each section is self contained, meaning you can jump around and needn't read in any kind of order to get the most of out of the recipes. Alternatively, dedicated aromatherapy enthusiasts can treat this book as a sequential guide, perhaps trying each recipe over the course of 200 days.

Each essential oil recipe is formulated for use with a cool mist diffuser, ideally Radha Beauty's model (more on why below) . You should not attempt to repurpose the recipes in this book for use with candles, teas, humidifiers, or any aromatherapy system other than a cool mist diffuser. At best, the benefits will be reduced; at worst, injuries or accidents could occur.

Used with a cool mist diffuser, all the recipes here are completely safe and maximally effective. All the blends are measured out for a cool mist diffuser with a 100 ml container capacity. Those using a diffuser with a different size of container should adjust the ratios accordingly.

COOL MIST DIFFUSION BASICS

Designed to emit micro-thin vapors, a good cool mist diffuser will produce the most benefit while using the least amount of those precious essential oils. Vaporizers, humidifiers and other warm air diffusers require heating, which can break down the oils and degrade them in the process, lessening their therapeutic effects.

Diffusers like Radha Beauty's also prevent the potential health risks associated with misuse of some oils. Certain plant extracts can be harmful if swallowed or administered directly to the skin, particularly in large or concentrated doses. Candles, tinctures, teas, and other aromatherapy delivery systems are inappropriate and possibly dangerous with the wrong substances. Used incorrectly, common and highly beneficial ingredients such as eucalyptus, nutmeg and wintergreen oil might produce rashes, internal irritations, or worse. Cool mist diffusion on the other hand, delivers all the benefits from these and other essential oils, with none of the risk.

Though there's no accounting for how every individual might react to every substance, and while you should avoid known allergens that have caused you trouble in the past, the tiny amounts of essential oil required for effective cool mist diffusion rule out most or all adverse reactions that may result from other aromatherapy methods.

WHAT'S SO GREAT ABOUT RADHA BEAUTY'S DIFFUSER?

Technically any cool mist diffuser would do fine for the recipes in this book, though they're not all created equal. I recommend Radha Beauty's product because it is the most versatile, high quality, user friendly model on the market.

I've personally used it to test every essential oil recipe in this book and then some. Radha's diffuser is fully portable, weighing in at only 11 ounces, and comes with a super long 6-foot power cord. You can set it to operate at a "continuous mist" mode, or for 30-seconds-on/30-seconds-off segments at "intermittent mist" mode.

Powerful enough to fill a space of 150 square feet with the aromas of your choice, it automatically shuts off when the water is empty, for added safety and energy efficiency. It also comes with the option of LED lighting in seven different colors and like all of Radha's products, it's made from all natural materials, for a holistic experience from start to finish.

At its capacity of 100 ml, the Radha Beauty diffuser will work for three hours in continuous mode, or six hours in intermittent mode. Thanks to its ultrasonic technology, Radha Beauty's diffuser is also the most silent on the market. Hooray for cool mist, AND *quiet* mist!

While some diffusers aren't made to handle continuous usage or the addition of certain ingredients, Radha's holds up brilliantly in every instance, no

matter the ingredients or desired duration. Readers employing another brand
of cool mist diffuser should first read the manufacturer's instructions
and product details, to ensure correct usage.

PROPER STORAGE OF ESSENTIAL OILS

Pure, undiluted essential oils have no 'expiration date'. But time, sunlight, and oxidation – which happens every time we open the bottle – even-
tually degrade the oils and diminish their therapeutic properties. The
shelf lives of essential oils vary depending on the type of plant and
its properties, as well as the methods that were used to distill or
extract the oils.

If stored correctly, most pure essential oils should stay fresh for at
least a year, even with regular use. But some compounds are more stable
than others, and it's always a good idea to mark the date you purchased
a given product on the bottle, so you can keep track of how long you've
had it and when it might be time to restock.

To preserve freshness as long as possible, store essential oils in
darkly colored glass bottles (amber and cobalt are most common), with
tightly sealed lids, in a cool, dark, dry place. Some aromatherapists
advise refrigerating essential oils, though it's not necessary. Never
store essential oils in plastic containers, which are easily corroded by
the oils' compounds.

HEALTH AND SAFETY TIPS BEFORE YOU GET STARTED

Along with avoiding any ingredients to which you're personally allergic, you should also check with your family members, roommates, co-workers, or whoever else will be exposed to the cool mist diffusion of a given recipe. One person's sweet fennel digestive aid may be another person's red eyed sneezing fit.

Though allergic reactions are extremely rare in cool mist diffusion, even trace amounts of certain substances could be harmful to those who are particularly sensitive, especially over prolonged periods of time. Be sure to ask all co-occupants about their allergies and intolerances, and steer clear of ingredients that might cause them trouble. Those who experience epileptic seizures, chronic heart disease, or other conditions, may be at specific risk and should consult their physicians before using any aromatherapy methods.

As with all treatments and remedies, pregnant women should also check with their doctor or midwife before using aromatherapies. While many ingredients will be both safe and beneficial to expectant mothers, particularly when used with a cool mist diffuser, some essential oils may be inappropriate in certain conditions. The first trimester of pregnancy is a particularly sensitive period and pregnant women are advised to be especially cautious with any substances inhaled or ingested.

WHAT ABOUT THE PETS?

Dogs, horses, and other pets often enjoy the benefits of essential oil aromatherapy along with their human companions. But, just like people, all animals are different and some may be sensitive to a given ingredient. If your pet exhibits negative reactions to any ingredient or recipe — scratching or sneezing, throwing up, whining or moaning — stop using it immediately and consult a veterinarian if the reaction continues.

Cats are particularly sensitive — much more so than dogs, horses, or humans — and their toxicity levels are generally lower. Their metabolisms are built differently, and their livers lack the enzymes required to break down certain compounds. These compounds include phenols and hydrocarbons, which occur naturally in many essential oils and are easily processed by human metabolisms, but are potentially harmful to cats.

While it's unlikely that the low-dose exposures resulting from cool-mist diffusion will bother most felines, cat-owners should nonetheless proceed with caution and avoid using essential oils that are high in phenols and hydrocarbons. These include:

- Lemon
- Lime
- Orange
- Bergamot
- Tangerine
- Pine
- Mandarin
- Spruce
- Grapefruit
- Fir
- Cassia (cinnamon)
- Thyme
- Clove
- Savory
- Oregano
- Wintergreen
- Tea tree
- Eucalyptus

Regardless of the ingredients used, be sure to keep a close eye on all pets exposed to new substances until you're sure they aren't having an adverse reaction. For more information on plants and derivatives that are potentially harmful to cats in particular, the Cat Fanciers' Association provides extensive information on its website.

QUALITY MATTERS!

The rising popularity of essential oils and aromatherapy in recent years has drawn tons of new suppliers into the market. That's meant an explosion in new brands and choices for consumers, but it also means a lot of low quality products on the market.

Unscrupulous manufacturers will attempt to pass off synthetic substances as "all natural," or dilute their oils with chemicals that could have adverse reactions. Others employ sloppy quality control and don't take care to store products appropriately, nor to rotate stock often enough to guarantee freshness. It's important to stick to reputable essential oil sellers, and to do one's research before trying out new brands. Check out online reviews by experts and other customers, and be sure to read up on a company's sourcing and safety protocols.

One fast way to spot a shoddy essential oil product is by the packaging: Undiluted, pure essential oils should never be stored in plastic bottles, as they risk corroding the plastic. They also shouldn't be contained in clear glass bottles, since they require protection from direct sunlight. High quality essential oils will always be packaged in dark colored glass bottles, usually amber or cobalt.

Little surprise, I am a huge fan of Radha Beauty's line of essential oils, all 100% pure and therapeutic grade. Other highly regarded essential oil brands include Young Living™, dōTERRA®, and Edens Gardens™. When in doubt, consult a naturopath, masseuse or holistic therapist you trust for recommendations on the best products for your needs.

MIND

Memory, Focus, Clarity, Alertness, and Concentration

The mind is an incredible organ — part machine and part deity, creator of art and science, processor of memories and knowledge and understanding. The possibilities of our minds are literally limitless, and when they are operating at their best, there is no telling what we can accomplish.

The recipes in this section contain powerful combinations of essential oils whose properties are known to stimulate, enhance, and support the key mental functions that make us great. From the extract of hyssop, which refreshes and energizes synaptic connections, to the clarifying and focus-friendly oil of the vetiver plant, essential oils can be highly effective in refining and optimizing mental properties.

Whether you're looking to get the most out of a team at work, or trying to create the ideal atmosphere for studying or for creative work, there's a recipe in here to help. The right aromatic blend can support both clear and enlightened thinking, and support the entire nervous and emotional system in creating the most conducive states for learn-ing and processing.

There is no secret to intellectual or artistic greatness — each of us possesses that potential inside of us. The challenge is to get the most of what we've already got in these wondrous brains of ours — and these recipes are a great place to start.

WAKE-UP ZINGER

This is a terrific recipe for first thing in the morning, when you need your brain working quickly and clearly. The peppermint and cinnamon are better than all the coffee in the world for stimulating your mind and inspiring creativity, while the touch of rosemary helps maintain calm and focus.

Ingredients:

★ 4 drops of peppermint oil

★ 4 drops of cinnamon oil

★ 2 drops of rosemary oil

★ 100 ml of water

Instructions: Fill the diffuser container with fresh water (straight from the tap, or distilled or filtered, depending on preference). Add the drops of peppermint, cinnamon, and rosemary, then plug in the diffuser and turn it on at the desired setting.

For additional consideration: Even if you're not a morning person, this blend will make you feel like one. Breathe deeply, enjoy, and greet the new day with a smile!

MARVELOUS MORNING

Here's another recipe that's ideal for the A.M. Simple and invigorating, the combined aromas of wild orange and peppermint are as bright and refreshing as sunlight itself. This citrus-rich blend is an especially good recipe to use during the cold, dark winter months, when everyone could use a warm picker-upper in the mornings.

Ingredients:

★ 4 drops of wild orange oil
★ 4 drops of peppermint oil
★ 100 ml of water

Instructions: Fill the diffuser container with fresh water (straight from the tap, or distilled or filtered, depending on preference). Add the drops of wild orange and peppermint, then plug in the diffuser and turn it on at the desired setting.

For additional consideration: It won't take long to warm up with this seasonal mix. Let the sweet, rich aromas fill the room and awaken your senses and your mind.

ADHD AID

Attention deficit and hyperactivity disorder, commonly known as ADHD, can be a serious impediment to children and young adults attempting to focus and accomplish mental tasks. The oils in this blend have been scientifically demonstrated to improve scholastic performance, and is particularly effective in children between the ages of 6 and 12 years.

Ingredients:

★ 4 drops of cedarwood oil
★ 2 drops of lavender oil
★ 2 drops of vetiver oil
★ 100 ml of water

Instructions: Fill the diffuser container with fresh water (straight from the tap, or distilled or filtered, depending on preference). Add the drops of cedarwood, lavender, and vetiver oil, then plug in the diffuser and turn it on at the desired setting.

For additional consideration: This is a great blend to help calm and focus the mind, and improve concentration for anyone who struggles with it during mental tasks. With a few deep breaths, this blend will have the mental faculties stimulated and working at their best.

CLARIFYING SUNSHINE

This is an excellent blend to freshen your thoughts and brighten your mood in the mornings or early afternoons, when everyone could use a calming but energizing pick-me-up. This stimulating blend of peppermint, lemon and frankincense is a great way to inject some vitality into your day — and it's a great alternative to that morning cup of coffee!

Ingredients:

★ 4 drops of peppermint oil
★ 2 drops of frankincense oil
★ 4 drops of lemon
★ 100 ml of water

Instructions: Fill the diffuser container with fresh water (straight from the tap, or distilled or filtered, depending on preference). Add the drops of peppermint, lemon, and frankincense, then plug in the diffuser and turn it on at the desired setting.

For additional consideration: Breathe deeply and enjoy these refreshing, grounding aromas. Then get on with your day feeling clearer and more right of mind!

MEMORY MASTER

This blend packs the power duo of rosemary and tarragon, both excellent for improving overall mental function and specifically for helping stimulate the parts of the brain responsible for handling information. Mixed with some refreshing, uplifting lemon oil, this is a great recipe to use regularly to maintain sharpness.

Ingredients:

★ 3 drops of tarragon oil

★ 3 drops of lemon oil

★ 2 drops of rosemary oil

Instructions: Fill the diffuser container with fresh water (straight from the tap, or distilled or filtered, depending on preference). Add the drops of tarragon, lemon, and rosemary, then plug in the diffuser and turn it on at the desired setting.

For additional consideration: Take a moment to savor the rich, layered aroma, and don't be surprised if your day is a little more vivid and bright.

SMARTY-PANTS SCHOLAR

This is a fantastic blend to use while working or studying. The rosemary and frankincense nurture a calm and focused mind, ideal for improving memory, as well as accomplishing analytical and critical tasks. The peppermint will keep you alert and refreshed, which is particularly helpful for those assignments and tasks that last long into the night.

Ingredients:

★ 3 drops of rosemary oil
★ 3 drops of frankincense oil
★ 3 drops of peppermint oil
★ 100 ml of water

Instructions: Fill the diffuser container with fresh water (straight from the tap, or distilled or filtered, depending on preference). Add the drops of rosemary, frankincense, and peppermint, then plug in the diffuser and turn it on at the desired setting.

For additional consideration: This recipe works well for the home or the office - anyplace that you want your mind at its most fertile. Prepare to feel invigorated and primed for your best work!

MIND-MASTER MELD

This blend uses the oil from the glorious vetiver plant, better known as khus in its native India. Its medicinal and therapeutic properties have been known to South Asian healers for millennia. The oil of the vetiver root helps to raise energy levels in moments of exhaustion, it also works to cool the body in moments of stress or tension. In Sri Lanka, its extract is known as the "oil of tranquility." Mingled with the calming properties of frankincense, this simple recipe is great for aiding concentration and focus.

Ingredients:
★ 4 drops of vetiver oil
★ 4 drops of frankincense
★ 100 ml of water

Instructions: Fill the diffuser container with fresh water (straight from the tap, or distilled or filtered, depending on preference). Add the drops of vetiver and frankincense, then plug in the diffuser and turn it on at the desired setting.

For additional consideration: The properties in this blend are also known to soothe anxiety and decrease attention deficits. Sit back and take in the restorative aroma that will clear your mind and sharpen your thinking.

GRANDMA'S
LITTLE HELPER

This recipe is an old classic, and for good reason. A hint of lemon and a slightly -bigger hint of rosemary will concentrate the mind and settle the nerves. It couldn't be simpler, and it works every time to add a sense of productive calm to any space.

Ingredients:

★ 5 drops of rosemary oil
★ 3 drops of lemon oil
★ I00 ml of water

Instructions: Fill the diffuser container with fresh water (straight from the tap, or distilled or filtered, depending on preference). Add the drops of rosemary and lemon, then plug in the diffuser and turn it on at the desired setting.

For additional consideration: This blend never fails to improve reasoning and intellect. As you breathe it in, take pleasure in knowing that you're inhaling the same aromas that people have used for millennia to sharpen their thinking.

PRODUCTIVITY POTION

This recipe is terrific when you can assemble all the ingredients, and creates the perfect aroma to have on continuous or intermittent mist during a busy day. The citrus zest of lemon and grapefruit, combined with an energizing dose of peppermint and basil, are perfectly balanced by the calming lavender and memory-boosting rosemary aromas.

Ingredients:

★ 1 drop of basil oil
★ 1 drop of rosemary oil
★ 2 drops of lemon oil
★ 100 ml of water

★ 2 drops of peppermint oil
★ 2 drops of grapefruit oil
★ 2 drops of lavender oil

Instructions: Fill the diffuser container with fresh water (straight from the tap, or distilled or filtered, depending on preference). Add the drops of basil, rosemary, lemon, peppermint, grapefruit, and lavender, then plug in the diffuser and turn it on at the desired setting.

For additional consideration: You're a few breaths away from a sustained surge of energy, without the edge! Relax and enjoy - there's no downside to this all-natural high.

PEACEFUL PEP

This recipe combines the energizing zing of grapefruit, lemon and basil with the calming serenity of lavender. These aromas go great together in just about any setting, producing an uplifting yet soothing scent that will keep your mind active and focused.

Ingredients:

★ 4 drops of grapefruit oil

★ 2 drops of lavender oil

★ 2 drops of lemon oil

★ 1 drop of basil oil

★ 100 ml of water

Instructions: Fill the diffuser container with fresh water (straight from the tap, or distilled or filtered, depending on preference). Add the drops of grapefruit, lavender, lemon and basil, then plug in the diffuser and turn it on at the desired setting.

For additional consideration: The combined aromas in this concentration-friendly blend work wonderfully in a home or office setting. Because of its energizing properties, this recipe is best for daytime use.

CLARITY CLEANSE

Tea-tree oil — also known as melaleuca — helps purify both the mind and the body, helping to clear everything from toxins to negative thoughts. Combined with lemon and lime in this refreshing recipe, the tea-tree oil is at its most effective, creating an ideal atmosphere for clear thinking.

Ingredients:

★ 3 drops of tea-tree oil
★ 3 drops of lemon oil
★ 3 drops of lime oil
★ 100 ml of water

Instructions: Fill the diffuser container with fresh water (straight from the tap, or distilled or filtered, depending on preference). Add the drops of tea-tree, lemon, and lime, then plug in the diffuser and turn it on at the desired setting.

For additional consideration: It's hard not to smile as you take your first inhales of this refreshing diffusion. Don't be surprised if you soon find yourself in a relaxed and enlightened state!

FOCUS FACTOR

The wonderful vetiver plant is unmatched in its soothing properties. A calm mind is a retentive mind, making this oil an excellent ingredient to use while analyzing data or committing facts to memory. With the bracing lemon and playful peppermint to maximize alertness, this is another great recipe for studying, writing, or focusing on just about any mental task.

Ingredients:
★ 4 drops of vetiver oil
★ 2 drops of lemon oil
★ 2 drops of peppermint oil
★ 100 ml of water

Instructions: Fill the diffuser container with fresh water (straight from the tap, or distilled or filtered, depending on preference). Add the drops of vetiver, lemon, and peppermint, then plug in the diffuser and turn it on at the desired setting.

For additional consideration: This is a tried-and-true favorite for keeping the mind settled and productive. The subtle but powerful aromas will start concentrating your thinking right away.

FOCUS ON FIRE

Need to concentrate as you've never concentrated before? This blend is for those days when you need to think like a superhero, with the powerful zing of orange and peppermint creating a power-duo to jumpstart your mental stamina and memory retention.

Ingredients:
★ 4 drops of orange oil
★ 4 drops of peppermint oil
★ 100 ml of water

Instructions: Fill the diffuser container with fresh water (straight from the tap, or distilled or filtered, depending on preference). Add the drops of orange and peppermint, then plug in the diffuser and turn it on at the desired setting.

For additional consideration: This stimulating and energizing blend will increase your mental alertness and help you to focus like a laser beam on whatever task is in front of you. Breathe deeply, and get ready to start thinking at your very best!

FEED YOUR HEAD

No, not in the "go ask Alice" druggy sense - in the all-natural, essential oil sense, that is! This excellent blend of eucalyptus, peppermint, and basil is serious nourishment for the mind - the perfect way to ward off mental fatigue and help give yourself everything you need for an enriched, powerful headspace.

Ingredients:
★ 4 drops of eucalyptus oil
★ 2 drops of peppermint oil
★ 2 drops of basil oil
★ 100 ml of water

Instructions: Fill the diffuser container with fresh water (straight from the tap, or distilled or filtered, depending on preference). Add the drops of eucalyptus, peppermint, and basil, then plug in the diffuser and turn it on at the desired setting.

For additional consideration: Use this blend any time you feel mental fatigue taking hold and you need to carry on. Breathe deeply and let this re- freshing aromatic combination give you the mental boost you need to see you through.

SIMPLY CENTERED

This is a simple recipe that's easy to make anytime you want to create an uplifting and grounded atmosphere. Extract from the cypress plant is one of the best oils around to foster a sense of mental stability and well-being, while the uplifting aroma of spearmint oil will help increase calm alertness.

Ingredients:

★ 3 drops of cypress oil
★ 3 drops of spearmint oil
★ 100 ml of water

Instructions: Fill the diffuser container with fresh water (straight from the tap, or distilled or filtered, depending on preference). Add the drops of cypress and spearmint, then plug in the diffuser and turn it on at the desired setting.

For additional consideration: This is a great recipe to enjoy in your diffuser any time of day, in just about any setting, so relax and breathe happy! You're unlikely to get anything but thanks from those sharing the space with you.

COOL HEADS

The purifying properties of tea-tree oil balance beautifully with the extract of the cilantro plant, which is known to reduce stress and actively cool down the body. With the addition of lemon and lime, they combine to create this clean, refreshing blend that will foster calm and clear thinking — you, at your best.

Ingredients:
★ 3 drops of lemon oil
★ 2 drops of tea-tree oil
★ 2 drops of cilantro oil
★ 2 drops of lime oil
★ 100 ml of water

Instructions: Fill the diffuser container with fresh water (straight from the tap, or distilled or filtered, depending on preference).Add the drops of lemon, tea-tree, cilantro, and lime, then plug in the diffuser and turn it on at the desired setting.

For additional consideration: Let the aroma fill your space and relax your mind. This blend will also have a cleansing and detoxifying effect on the body and spirit, for a truly holistic diffusion experience.

UP AND AT 'EM

Hyssop oil is a safe and effective stimulant, and an excellent overall tonic for the entire nervous system. Mingled with the cleansing and restorative aroma of lemon, it makes this an easy recipe for an all-around mental pick-me-up. This blend is terrific for fostering concentration and focus, while maintaining calm and easing stress.

Ingredients:

★ 3 drops of hyssop oil

★ 3 drops of lemon oil

★ 100 ml of water

Instructions: Fill the diffuser container with fresh water (straight from the tap, or distilled or filtered, depending on preference). Add the drops of hyssop and lemon, then plug in the diffuser and turn it on at the desired setting.

For additional consideration: The hyssop and lemon in this recipe are also effective detoxifiers for the whole body, along with their rejuvenating effects on the mind. Enjoy this happy, energizing aroma any time of the day or night.

PEACE OF MIND

This beautiful blend contains everything you need to create a sooth-ing, serene setting. Lavender oil is well-known to settle anxiety, and is only enhanced by the calming, restorative properties of rosemary and peppermint. Thyme and marjoram are both effective tonics for the nerves, and marjoram has been known to act as both a pain-killer and a sedative.

Ingredients:

★ 2 drops of marjoram oil
★ 2 drops of rosemary oil
★ 2 drops of lavender oil
★ 2 drops of thyme oil
★ 2 drops of peppermint oil
★ 100 ml of water

Instructions: Fill the diffuser container with fresh water (straight from the tap, or distilled or filtered, depending on preference). Add the drops of marjoram, thyme, rosemary, peppermint, and lavender, then plug in the diffuser and turn it on at the desired setting.

For additional consideration: Breathing in these aromas is often found to help ease headaches, along with producing a more general sense of men-tal well-being A few deep inhales, and your head will be in good shape.

GROUNDED MIND

This blend supports emotional stability and wise decision-making. The basil and hyssop are a wonderful duo for stimulating your mental retention and information processing, while the lavender will calm your nerves and keep your thinking supple.

Ingredients:

★ 3 drops of hyssop oil

★ 3 drops of lavender oil

★ 2 drops of basil oil

★ 100 ml of water

Instructions: Fill the diffuser container with fresh water (straight from the tap, or distilled or filtered, depending on preference). Add the drops of hyssop, lavender, and basil, then plug in the diffuser and turn it on at the desired setting. This is a wonderful blend to use at midday, or anytime in the afternoon or evening.

TERRIFIC TRAVELER

Got a long road trip or plane ride coming up? Before you set off, give yourself the aromatic antidote to all the frantic, last-minute chaos that precedes a long voyage with a relaxing and refreshing blend. The lavender, clary sage, geranium and peppermint in this recipe are the perfect tonic to reinvigorate you both physically and emotionally, and energize you for the road ahead.

Ingredients:

★ 3 drops of lavender oil
★ 2 drops of clary sage oil
★ IOO ml of water
★ 2 drops of peppermint oil
★ I drops of geranium oil

Instructions: Fill the diffuser container with fresh water (straight from the tap, or distilled or filtered, depending on preference). Add the drops of lavender, clary sage, geranium, and peppermint, then plug in the diffuser and turn it on at the desired setting.

For additional consideration: A few deep breaths of blend, and you'll feel primed and ready for your trip — come what may! Focused, refreshed, and ready to go, there's nothing left to do but *bon voyage!*

ELEVATED MIND

The happy yellow inula flower has been used for centuries for its restorative properties. Its oil's aroma is thought to stimulate mental retention and information processing, and the cheerful floral scent mingles perfectly with grounding laurel and cleansing grapefruit in this fresh, uplifting blend.

Ingredients:

★ 3 drops of inula oil

★ 3 drops of laurel oil

★ 2 drops of grapefruit oil

★ 100 ml of water

Instructions: Fill the diffuser container with fresh water (straight from the tap, or distilled or filtered, depending on preference). Add the drops of inula, laurel, and grapefruit, then plug in the diffuser and turn it on at the desired setting.

For additional consideration: This recipe will quickly enrich your mind and, in turn, lift your spirits. Enjoy this blend any time of day or night, and let it bring your intellect to new heights.

MENTAL REJUVENATION

The humble strawflower is known to healers and aestheticians as "immortelle," or the "everlasting daisy." In this recipe it works with the intellect-stimulating frankincense oil and a hint of eucalyptus to refresh the mind and restore sharpness and clarity to your thoughts.

Ingredients:

★ 3 drops of strawflower oil

★ 3 drops of frankincense oil

★ 1 drop of eucalyptus oil

Instructions: Fill the diffuser container with fresh water (straight from the tap, or distilled or filtered, depending on preference). Add the drops of strawflower, frankincense, and eucalyptus, then plug in the diffuser and turn it on at the desired setting.

For additional consideration: Breathe deeply and feel yourself grow energized and inspired. This is an excellent blend to use at midday to maintain focused mental momentum.

SO SERENE

This recipe is an excellent mix to diffuse during a meditation or yoga session. The cedarwood scent is both calming and uplifting, and ylang-ylang oil is well known as a powerful stress-reliever and overall nervous-system booster. With a high ratio of soothing lavender, and just enough wild orange to sweeten your senses and keep the mind alert, this blend will bring deep and productive serenity to any space.

Ingredients:

★ 4 drops of lavender oil
★ 2 drops of wild orange oil
★ 2 drops of cedarwood oil
★ I drop of ylang-ylang oil
★ IOO ml of water

Instructions: Fill the diffuser container with fresh water (straight from the tap, or distilled or filtered, depending on preference). Add the drops of lavender, wild orange, cedarwood, and ylang ylang, then plug in the diffuser and turn it on at the desired setting.

For additional consideration: This blend will contribute to heightened awareness and overall well-being. A few deep breaths, and your head will be in good shape.

COOL HEADS PREVAIL

This is an excellent blend to diffuse on those days when you're feeling a little hot under the collar — or when you could simply use a cooling, cleansing atmosphere on a warm day. The combination of lavender, spearmint and peppermint is both calming and invigorating — perfect to put and keep you in your coolest head!

Ingredients:
- ★ 3 drops of lavender oil
- ★ 2 drops of spearmint oil
- ★ 2 drops of peppermint oil
- ★ 100 ml of water

Instructions: Fill the diffuser container with fresh water (straight from the tap, or distilled or filtered, depending on preference). Add the drops of lavender, peppermint, and spearmint, then plug in the diffuser and turn it on at the desired setting.

For additional consideration: This minty, floral blend will have your mind feeling cooler and clearer in no time. This blend is fine to use any time of day — invigorating enough for mornings, but calming and stabilizing enough for the evenings or before bedtime. Just breathe deeply, and enjoy those cool, clear thoughts!

MENTAL BALANCE

This beautiful blend is the perfect mixture to help clear your mind, focus your thoughts, and keep life in perspective - whatever the day may bring. The combination of rose, orange, and vetiver oil is perfect for those moments when you're feeling frazzled or confused, and will help restore mental equilibrium and a deep sense of clarity.

Ingredients:

★ 3 drops of orange oil   ★ 2 drops of rose oil

★ 1 drop of vetiver oil   ★ 100 ml of water

Instructions: Fill the diffuser container with fresh water (straight from the tap, or distilled or filtered, depending on preference). Add the drops of rose, orange, and vetiver, then plug in the diffuser and turn it on at the desired setting.

For additional consideration: Let this lovely mixture of floral and woody aromas with citrus overtones refresh your mind, clear your thoughts, and restore balance to your day. With a few deep breaths, you'll be feeling more centered in no time - ready to take on any challenge with wisdom and calm.

CLEAR CONFIDENCE

Juniper berry oil is a wonderful support for both the mind and spirit. Its sweet, musky aroma is both comforting and galvanizing, and combines here with lemon and lavender for a refreshing, calming mix that's sure to help everyone who breathes it to put their best foot forward.

Ingredients:

★ 3 drops of juniper berry oil

★ 3 drops of lemon oil

★ 3 drops of lavender oil

★ 100 ml of water

Instructions: Fill the diffuser container with fresh water (straight from the tap, or distilled or filtered, depending on preference). Add the drops of juniper berry, lemon and lavender, then plug in the diffuser and turn it on at the desired setting.

For additional consideration: These aromas are effective and longlasting - and their beneficial properties take action fast. Don't be shocked if, after a few breaths, you find yourself thinking happier thoughts for the rest of the day.

ULTIMATE CLARITY

This powerful blend of oils is one of the most effective recipes out there for clearing the mind and soothing the body. It combines the uplifting properties of lemon and peppermint with the calming aromas of bergamot and jasmine, to produce a balanced but potent blend for mental sharpness and overall well-being.

Ingredients:

★ 3 drops of lemon oil
★ 3 drops of jasmine oil
★ 2 drops of peppermint oil
★ 2 drops of bergamot oil
★ 100 ml of water

Instructions: Fill the diffuser container with fresh water (straight from the tap, or distilled or filtered, depending on preference). Add the drops of lemon, jasmine, peppermint, and bergamot, then plug in the diffuser and turn it on at the desired setting.

For additional consideration: There is no drug that can compare to the exhilaration of true clarity and inner enlightenment. Enjoy the all-natural and restorative effects of this serene blend.

CREATIVITY TONIC

Got a creative project that needs your absolute best faculties? This stimulating blend of energizing and uplifting aromas is perfect to inspire you and get those creative juices flowing, helping you to produce your absolute best work.

Ingredients:
* ★ 2 drops of basil oil
* ★ 2 drops of ylang-ylang oil
* ★ I drop of petitgrain oil
* ★ 2 drops of rosemary oil
* ★ I drop of cardamom oil
* ★ IOO ml of water

Instructions: Fill the diffuser container with fresh water (straight from the tap, or distilled or filtered, depending on preference). Add the drops of basil, rosemary, ylang-ylang, cardamom, and petitgrain, then plug in the diffuser and turn it on at the desired setting.

For additional consideration: Whether you've got an art project that needs to be truly special, or simply a problem at work or home that needs creative thinking, this is a wonderful blend to diffuse and put yourself at your very best. A few deep breaths and you'll start seeing solutions where before there were none. So inhale, exhale, and get going with a smile!

INSPIRATION FROM THE INSIDE

This is another great blend for those moments when you need to be at your creative best. The ho wood essential oil is a powerful fragrance that will stimulate relaxation and emotional fluidity, while the clary sage, patchouli and pine oil in this blend will help set it off and maintain clear, focused thinking.

Ingredients:

★ 3 drops of ho wood oil

★ 2 drops of clary sage oil

★ 2 drops of pine oil

★ 1 drop of patchouli oil

★ 100 ml of water

Instructions: Fill the diffuser container with fresh water (straight from the tap, or distilled or filtered, depending on preference). Add the drops of ho wood, clary sage, pine oil, and patchouli, then plug in the diffuser and turn it on at the desired setting.

For additional consideration: Whether you're feeling well and truly blocked on a task, or just looking to kick-start your next project, this is a delightful "daydreamy" blend to get your ideas flowing. Breathe deeply and let yourself be inspired!

WISE OWL

This recipe is fantastic for work or study sessions. The powerful combination of focus-inducing rosemary, juniper berry and tea-tree oil will stimulate the mind and focus the thinking. This blend is best enjoyed in the morning, and is particularly helpful when tackling tough problems that require strong judgment.

Ingredients:

★ 3 drops of rosemary oil

★ 3 drops of juniper berry oil

★ 3 drops of tea-tree oil

★ 100 ml of water

Instructions: Fill the diffuser container with fresh water (straight from the tap, or distilled or filtered, depending on preference). Add the drops of rosemary, juniper berry, and tea tree, then plug in the diffuser and turn it on at the desired setting.

For additional consideration: After a few satisfying breaths of this balanced mix, you'll be ready for any challenge. This might be a great time to solve all the problems of the world! Or just take advantage of your mind at its most concentrated and wise state.

DECISION-MAKING ELIXIR

If you're one of those people who feels indecisive about even the smallest choices, or if you're simply having a hard time making up your mind on a single important question, this is the blend for you. The combination of basil, peppermint, lime and rosemary is the perfect way to wake up your mind and increase alertness and mental clarity, to make the best possible decision — whatever the question.

Ingredients:

★ 3 drops of basil oil
★ 2 drops of lime oil
★ 100 ml of water
★ 2 drops of peppermint oil
★ I drop of rosemary oil

Instructions: Fill the diffuser container with fresh water (straight from the tap, or distilled or filtered, depending on preference). Add the drops of basil, peppermint, lime, and rosemary, then plug in the diffuser and turn it on at the desired setting.

For additional consideration: This energizing blend will help to combat fatigue and stimulate alertness and clarity. Enjoy this blend any time you have a tough decision to make, and breathe deeply in the confidence that you're in your best mind to make a good choice.

PERSPECTIVE PLUS

When you've lost sight of what's important, or are having trouble letting go of negativity, this blend will help you to clear your mind and regain some much needed perspective.

Ingredients:

★ 4 drops of sandalwood oil

★ 2 drops of lavender oil

★ I drop of orange oil

★ IOO ml of water

Instructions: Fill the diffuser container with fresh water (straight from the tap, or distilled or filtered, depending on preference). Add the drops of sandalwood, lavender, and orange, then plug in the diffuser and turn it on at the desired setting.

For additional consideration: Enjoy the clarifying sense of balance and stability that comes with every breath of this blend. The sandalwood, lavender, and orange are the perfect way to right whatever is going on in your mind, so inhale deeply, relax, and enjoy.

BRAWNY BRAINS

This recipe packs a punch - an intellectual punch, that is, in the best possible way. Cedarwood and basil and perfectly matched with a hint of ginger and black pepper for a rich blend to stimulate sustained focus and mental clarity. This is a particularly good recipe for use in the workplace, as it's not too flowery.

Ingredients:

★ 4 drops of cedarwood oil   ★ 2 drops of basil oil

★ 1 drop of ginger oil   ★ 1 drop of black pepper oil

★ 100 ml of water

Instructions: Fill the diffuser container with fresh water (straight from the tap, or distilled or filtered, depending on preference). Add the drops of cedarwood, basil, ginger, and black pepper, then plug in the diffuser and turn it on at the desired setting.

For additional consideration: Breathe in and smile - your brain is getting primed for its very best work, and with this intellectually enriching diffusion, nothing can stand in your way.

CONCENTRATED CONCENTRATION

The juniper berry, pine, and rosemary essential oils in this blend are an excellent way to get your mind focused - and keep it that way. This is an excellent blend for any mental task that requires sustained concentration, so plug in and get going!

Ingredients:

★ 3 drops of juniper berry oil

★ 2 drops of pine oil

★ 2 drops of rosemary oil

★ 100 ml of water

Instructions: Fill the diffuser container with fresh water (straight from the tap, or distilled or filtered, depending on preference). Add the drops of juniper berry, pine, and rosemary, then plug in the diffuser and turn it on at the desired setting.

For additional consideration: After a few breaths of this focus-friendly blend, your mind will be ready to stop wandering and get on track. This is a subtle but powerful combination that is perfect to keep your attention where it is needed.

ALWAYS ALERT

You know those kung-fu masters in classic martial-arts movies — the ones who always seem perfectly aware of their surroundings? That's how this stimulating blend of geranium, ylang-ylang, sandalwood and vetiver will make you feel after a few deep breaths. At once calming and invigorating, these oils will maximize your physical senses and mental acuity.

Ingredients:
★ 2 drops of geranium oil
★ 2 drops of ylang-ylang oil
★ 2 drops of sandalwood oil
★ I drop of vetiver oil
★ IOO ml of water

Instructions: Fill the diffuser container with fresh water (straight from the tap, or distilled or filtered, depending on preference). Add the drops of geranium, ylang-ylang, sandalwood, and vetiver, then plug in the diffuser and turn it on at the desired setting.

For additional consideration: As the fragrant aromas fill your space and your senses, relax into calm, productive alertness. This is a wonderful state for everyone from executives to creatives and management alike.

BRAIN BOOST

The combination of rosemary, cypress, and juniper berry is an excellent blend to wake up your mind and stimulate your best thinking. Need some powerful ideas or sustained focus? This is the blend for you.

Ingredients:

★ 2 drops of rosemary oil

★ 2 drops of cypress oil

★ 2 drops of juniper berry oil

★ 100 ml of water

Instructions: Fill the diffuser container with fresh water (straight from the tap, or distilled or filtered, depending on preference). Add the drops of rosemary, cypress, and juniper berry, then plug in the diffuser and turn it on at the desired setting.

For additional consideration: This is an outstanding way to give your brain a boost, and prevent mental fatigue from causing you to make mistakes. Let this refreshing and stimulating blend wake up your mind and help you keep going with focus and excellence. This is a terrific blend to ward off the mid-afternoon blahs. The energizing aromas are mellow enough to use through the early evening, with no risk of making it difficult to sleep at night. A few deep breaths of this blend, and you'll feel refreshed and ready to finish the day strong!

REMEMBER THIS

The basil and rosemary in this blend are the perfect ways to stimulate your memory, while the lemon creates a cleansing and refreshing effect on the body as well as the mind. This blend may help to ward off age-related memory loss, as well as that day-to-day forgetfulness that plagues many of us at any age.

Ingredients:

★ 4 drops of lemon oil   ★ 3 drops of basil oil

★ 2 drops of rosemary oil   ★ 100 ml of water

Instructions: Fill the diffuser container with fresh water (straight from the tap, or distilled or filtered, depending on preference). Add the drops of lemon, basil, and rosemary, then plug in the diffuser and turn it on at the desired setting.

For additional consideration: This light, herbaceous blend will help promote concentration and clarity of thought, both of which are essential for optimizing memory retention. Breathe deeply and enjoy the sense of focus that will inhabit your mind - the best possible state for making and keeping memories.

HOMEWORK HELPER

If your kids are anything like mine, they might need a little extra help to get in the right headspace to buckle down and do their homework. This mentally stabilizing blend of rosemary and lemongrass is the perfect way to nudge them in that direction – without any need for nagging!

Ingredients:

★ 4 drops of rosemary oil

★ 2 drops of lemongrass oil

★ 100 ml of water

Instructions: Fill the diffuser container with fresh water (straight from the tap, or distilled or filtered, depending on preference). Add the drops of rosemary and lemongrass, then plug in the diffuser and turn it on at the desired setting.

For additional consideration: With this blend providing a little gentle aromatic encouragement, homework won't seem like such a drag. Plug in and watch as the aromas from the diffuser help to calm and focus your child's mind, putting them in the right headspace to tackle their assignments with concentration and calm.

EXAM TIME

There's nothing like vetiver oil to stimulate the mind and focus the thinking. Mixed with concentration-friendly cedarwood and clarifying peppermint in this aromatic blend, and you've got the perfect diffusion to breathe in ahead of an exam, or any other task that requires your absolute best thinking.

Ingredients:
★ 3 drops of cedarwood oil
★ 2 drops of vetiver oil
★ 2 drops of peppermint oil
★ 100 ml of water

Instructions: Fill the diffuser container with fresh water (straight from the tap, or distilled or filtered, depending on preference). Add the drops of cedarwood, vetiver, and peppermint, then plug in the diffuser and turn it on at the desired setting.

For additional consideration: Breathe in this blend before setting off to sit your next exam — literally, or figuratively — and take a moment to relax and inhale these aromas. This blend will help calm your nerves and balance your mind, helping you to focus on whatever the task is at hand.

STUDY AID

This is another powerful blend to help your kids be in their best head-space for homework and study — or for adults that could use a little extra help focusing their minds. The rosemary, basil, and juniper berry oils are wonderful to improve memory retention, and the peppermint and clary sage provide just the kick you need to think clearly.

Ingredients:
★ 2 drops of rosemary oil
★ 2 drops of juniper berry oil
★ 2 drops of clary sage oil
★ 2 drops of basil oil
★ 2 drops of peppermint oil
★ 100 ml of water

Instructions: Fill the diffuser container with fresh water (straight from the tap, or distilled or filtered, depending on preference). Add the drops of rosemary, basil, juniper berry, peppermint, and clary sage, then plug in the diffuser and turn it on at the desired setting.

For additional consideration: Before study or homework time begins, take a few moments to close your eyes — or instruct your children or other scholars to do so — and breathe in this powerful blend. With just a few inhales, the mind will feel clearer and more focused, ready to learn and retain information. Breathe smart!

MIND FRESHENER

---★---

This recipe is a godsend for anyone stuck in a mental or creative rut. Struggling over complex data, or a persistent case of writers' block? Maybe you're having a hard time reorganizing that closet, or find yourself uninspired for a new design assignment? Never fear, this perfect blend of rosemary, basil, and Roman chamomile essential oils is here. This simple mix is both stimulating and mellow, and works great day or night to refresh your thinking.

Ingredients:

★ 3 drops of Roman chamomile oil
★ 2 drops of basil oil
★ 2 drops of rosemary oil
★ 100 ml of water

Instructions: Fill the diffuser container with fresh water (straight from the tap, or distilled or filtered, depending on preference). Add the drops of Roman chamomile, basil and rosemary, then plug in the diffuser and turn it on at the desired setting.

For additional consideration: Close your eyes and take a few deep breaths; open your eyes and enjoy seeing the world a little bit differently, anew.

SOOTHING SAGACITY

The elemi plant is from the same family as frankincense, and its soft, spicy aroma is a wonderful enhancement for a calm mind and steady mental state. With the concentration-friendly scent of rosemary and soothing touch of lavender, this is a wonderful recipe to stimulate clear thinking and rational decision-making.

Ingredients:

★ 3 drops of elemi oil

★ 3 drops of rosemary oil

★ 2 drops of lavender oil

★ 100 ml of water

Instructions: Fill the diffuser container with fresh water (straight from the tap, or distilled or filtered, depending on preference). Add the drops of elemi, rosemary and lavender, then plug in the diffuser and turn it on at the desired setting.

For additional consideration: Take a few slow inhales, and let the rich aromas unlock your best thinking. The clarifying energy that comes with this balanced diffusion is too good to miss.

WISE THREE

It's little surprise that the Three Wise Men in the Bible were packing frankincense and myrrh. The combination of these oils along with clarifying, enlightening tea tree oil is, effectively, the holy trinity of aromatherapeutic wisdom. Use any time of day or night, enjoying the harmonious scents and the elevated state of mind they bring.

Ingredients:
★ 3 drops frankincense oil
★ 3 drops myrrh oil
★ 3 drops tea-tree oil
★ 100 ml of water

Instructions: Fill the diffuser container with fresh water (straight from the tap, or distilled or filtered, depending on preference). Add the drops of frankincense, myrrh, and tea tree, then plug in the diffuser and turn it on at the desired setting.

For additional consideration: This is an excellent blend to use for special occasions (and you might want to, since myrrh is not cheap), or any time you want to add a touch of divinity to your thinking.

SMARTY SPICE

This is a fun and invigorating blend that kids will love along with adults. (Ssh, don't tell them it's probably also helping them excel at their homework!) The cinnamon and nutmeg give a playful but focus-friendly zing to a space, while the tea-tree oil works its power on nurturing mental strength and sustained concentration.

Ingredients:
- ★ 5 drops of tea-tree oil
- ★ 2 drops of cinnamon oil
- ★ 2 drops of nutmeg oil
- ★ 100 ml of water

Instructions: Fill the diffuser container with fresh water (straight from the tap, or distilled or filtered, depending on preference). Add the drops of tea tree, cinnamon, and nutmeg, then plug in the diffuser and turn it on at the desired setting.

For additional consideration: Everyone loves the mellow spice of this blend, so don't hesitate to use it in the office as well as the home. Let the aromas fill whatever space you're in, and enrich your thinking throughout the day.

SUPERBRAIN POWER BLEND

Prepare to be invigorated! This recipe is absolute dynamite - in the good way. The high ratio of restorative ylang-ylang, known to promote equilibrium and confidence, along with revitalizing cardamom oil, will help you operate at your very best. The rosewood and geranium contribute to support mental stability and overall calm, making this blend ideal for when you need a sustained intellectual boost.

Ingredients:

★ 3 drops of ylang-ylang oil
★ 2 drops of cardamom oil
★ 100 ml of water

★ 2 drops of rosewood oil
★ 2 drops of geranium oil

Instructions: Fill the diffuser container with fresh water (straight from the tap, or distilled or filtered, depending on preference). Add the drops of ylang-ylang, rosewood, cardamom, and geranium, then plug in the diffuser and turn it on at the desired setting.

For additional consideration: This blend has a way of fostering intellectual super-heroism. Before you know it, you'll have summoned your own inner Einstein!

AWESOME AWARENESS

This is a terrific blend to help achieve that state of mind where you're both fully alert and completely relaxed. It's mellow enough to use in the evenings, but more than effective enough to replace the morning coffee routine. Basil, melissa, lime and juniper berry extracts are an excellent blend to have in a home or office space, and a welcome addition to any focused thoughtflow.

Ingredients:
- ★ 3 drops of lime oil
- ★ 2 drops of melissa oil
- ★ 100 ml of water
- ★ 2 drops of juniper berry oil
- ★ 1 drop of basil oil

Instructions: Fill the diffuser container with fresh water (straight from the tap, or distilled or filtered, depending on preference). Add the drops of lime, juniper berry, melissa, and basil, then plug in the diffuser and turn it on at the desired setting.

For additional consideration: This is such a happy blend, that lends a truly joyful atmosphere to your mental state. Let the mist surround you like a calming, cheerful companion throughout the day.

SOOTHING MENTAL STRENGTH

Here's another recipe that will be a welcome addition to any yoga or meditation practice. The extracts of the citrus petitgrain are an exceptionally effective nerve tonic, known to help repair and strengthen the nervous system as a whole. The sweet floral aroma of the palmarosa oil is similarly restorative, and works in harmony with the lavender, cedarwood, and vetiver oils to promote sustained mental acuity and stability.

Ingredients:

★ 4 drops of lavender oil

★ 2 drops of cedarwood oil

★ I drop of vetiver oil

★ 2 drops of petitgrain oil

★ I drop of palmarosa oil

★ IOO ml of water

Instructions: Fill the diffuser container with fresh water (straight from the tap, or distilled or filtered, depending on preference). Add the drops of lavender, petitgrain, cedarwood, palmarosa, and vetiver, then plug in the diffuser and turn it on at the desired setting.

For additional consideration: Relax and feel your mind grow stronger and your thinking clearer. Your body and spirit will thank you too, as this blend helps you release tensions and absorb positive energy.

STEADY FLOW

The cheering properties of lemongrass oil work great with that perennial mental optimizer, rosemary, in this easy yet effective recipe. The touch of geranium oil lends an additional, restorative calm to the space, making this blend perfect for days when you need sustained and steady thought.

Ingredients:

★ 3 drops of lemongrass oil
★ 3 drops of rosemary oil
★ 2 drops of geranium oil
★ IOO ml of water

Instructions: Fill the diffuser container with fresh water (straight from the tap, or distilled or filtered, depending on preference). Add the drops of lemongrass, rosemary, and geranium, then plug in the diffuser and turn it on at the desired setting.

For additional consideration: Don't forget to savor the notes of each scent in this delicately balanced diffusion, as your mind focuses and your thinking clears.

SIMPLY BRILLIANT

This recipe is a winner every time, with relaxing rosewood balancing out the energizing tea-tree oil. Lavender evens out this blend for a mellow, clear aroma, creating an ideal atmosphere for clarity of thought and action. This uplifting recipe is effective enough for mornings, but not too stimulating for evenings. Its…simply brilliant!

Ingredients:

★ 3 drops of tea-tree oil

★ 3 drops of rosewood oil

★ 2 drops of lavender oil

★ 100 ml of water

Instructions: Fill the diffuser container with fresh water (straight from the tap, or distilled or filtered, depending on preference). Add the drops of tea-tree, rosewood, and lavender, then plug in the diffuser and turn it on at the desired setting.

For additional consideration: After a few deep breaths of this invigorating mix, you may find a pleasant feeling in your head and neck - the feeling of your mental processes warming up!

ZEN MASTER

Like frankincense and rosemary, white-fir oil is an excellent ingredient to stimulate both concentration and relaxation. The bracing aroma of the white-fir oil is both empowering and soothing. This recipe mixes in refreshing lemon and lime, along with cleansing tea-tree oil and cilantro, to create the ultimate blend for sustained mental clarity, focus, and memory retention.

Ingredients:

★ 3 drops of white-fir oil   ★ 2 drops of lemon oil
★ 2 drops of tea-tree oil   ★ 1 drop of cilantro oil
★ 1 drop of lime oil   ★ 100 ml of water

Instructions: Fill the diffuser container with fresh water (straight from the tap, or distilled or filtered, depending on preference). Add the drops of white fir, lemon, tea-tree, cilantro, and lime, then plug in the diffuser and turn it on at the desired setting.

For additional consideration: Take several long inhales and close your eyes; expect to soon find yourself in a deep and pleasant meditative state.

SUPERIOR MIND

Rosemary and cedarwood work in tandem to unlock your mind's highest aptitudes, with their complimentary aromas stimulating memory retention and problem solving. This blend has the added restorative zest of peppermint, to wrap your space with an energizing lift that's perfect for putting you at your best.

Ingredients:

★ 3 drops of rosemary oil
★ 2 drops of cedarwood oil
★ 2 drops of peppermint oil
★ 100 ml of water

Instructions: Fill the diffuser container with fresh water (straight from the tap, or distilled or filtered, depending on preference). Add the drops of rosemary, cedarwood, and peppermint, then plug in the diffuser and turn it on at the desired setting.

For additional consideration: Don't be afraid to take lots of long, deep breaths — you'll want to, and with each one your mind will feel better and better!

CREATIVE CALM

There is no calm quite like 'sandalwood calm.' This essential oil known for its soothing and uplifting antidepressant properties has been used in traditional medicine since time immemorial. With the addition of restorative geranium oil and the relaxing extracts of lavender, bergamot and Roman chamomile, this recipe is designed to nurture that elusive mental state known as "flow," enhancing your artistic energies.

Ingredients:

★ 3 drops of sandalwood oil
★ 2 drops of bergamot oil
★ I drop of Roman chamomile oil
★ 2 drops of lavender oil
★ 2 drops of geranium oil
★ IOO ml of water

Instructions: Fill the diffuser container with fresh water (straight from the tap, or distilled or filtered, depending on preference). Add the drops of sandalwood, lavender, bergamot, geranium, and Roman chamomile, then plug in the diffuser and turn it on at the desired setting.

For additional consideration: Make sure to have your paintbrushes, musical instruments, and other fine-art supplies ready while diffusing this blend — you're about to feel very creative!

NERVES OF STEEL

When the going gets tough, the tough get to their essential oil cupboard. This recipe contains clary sage extract, an uplifting compound widely known for its benefits to the overall nervous system, as well as those and concentration power houses marjoram and ylang-ylang. For good measure and a sustained, lasting sense of calm, lavender balances the blend.

Ingredients:

★ 3 drops of clary sage oil

★ 2 drops of marjoram oil

★ 100 ml of water

★ 3 drops of lavender oil

★ 2 drops of ylang-ylang oil

Instructions: Fill the diffuser container with fresh water (straight from the tap, or distilled or filtered, depending on preference). Add the drops of clary sage, lavender, marjoram, and ylang-ylang, then plug in the diffuser and turn it on at the desired setting.

For additional consideration: Settle back and feel your own inner strength grow. This blend is most helpful when you want to remind yourself of just how resilient you really are.

WISDOM FOR THE WISE

Melissa oil is commonly known as "lemon balm," though it's a member of the mint family. Whatever you call this gentle, stabilizing plant extract, it's one of the best to use when you need to summon true wisdom. The grounding Melissa helps open up emotional and intellectual barriers and nurtures true insight. Mingled with soothing lavender and just a touch of ylang-ylang, this recipe is truly wisdom for the wise.

Ingredients:

★ 3 drops of melissa oil

★ 3 drops of lavender oil

★ 2 drops of ylang-ylang oil

★ 100 ml of water

Instructions: Fill the diffuser container with fresh water (straight from the tap, or distilled or filtered, depending on preference). Add the drops of melissa, lavender, and ylang-ylang, then plug in the diffuser and turn it on at the desired setting.

For additional consideration: This recipe effectively unlocks our best selves. Take a good long breath, and let your deepest wisdom flourish.

CONTEMPLATION

Cleansing lemon, uplifting spearmint, and focus-inducing cypress oil in this blend are a wonderful aroma mix to put your mind in the best possible place for sustained, powerful contemplation. You know how everyone's always saying to think before you act? If that's difficult advice for you to follow — as it is for me — this diffusion is a great jump-start.

Ingredients:
★ 3 drops of lemon oil
★ 2 drops of spearmint oil
★ 2 drops of cypress oil
★ 100 ml of water

Instructions: Fill the diffuser container with fresh water (straight from the tap, or distilled or filtered, depending on preference). Add the drops of lemon, spearmint, and cypress, then plug in the diffuser and turn it on at the desired setting.

For additional consideration: This is my go-to diffusion for anytime I need to think deeply about an issue or situation before making a decision. Even if it's just a regular day, I love having this blend in my diffuser to help calm my emotions and stimulate reflective thought — something I could always use more of!

FREE MIND

Sure, we all remember patchouli as the companion scent of college parties and hippy dazes. But it's time to give this savory, warm aroma a second sniff — and enjoy the relaxing and invigorating properties it brings to any space. Mingled with the cleansing and refreshing lemon oils and a touch of focus-friendly bergamot, this blend is perfect for when you want to let your imagination run free.

Ingredients:
★ 3 drops of patchouli oil
★ 3 drops of lemon oil
★ I drop of bergamot
★ IOO ml of water

Instructions: Fill the diffuser container with fresh water (straight from the tap, or distilled or filtered, depending on preference). Add the drops of patchouli, lemon and bergamot, then plug in the diffuser and turn it on at the desired setting.

For additional consideration: This blend is great any time of day, but particularly useful when your thinking needs a gentle pick-me-up in the afternoon.

ENLIGHTENMENT BLEND

---------------------★---------------------

This recipe is a simple but well-kept secret. Nothing beats the fresh woodsy scent of spruce and a touch of lime to clarify your thoughts and expand your mind. This recipe is an excellent one to use in any space whose inhabitants could use a mental uplift - at work or in the home, this blend helps the light shine in.

Ingredients:

★ 5 drops of spruce oil

★ 2 drops of lime oil

★ 100 ml of water

Instructions: Fill the diffuser container with fresh water (straight from the tap, or distilled or filtered, depending on preference). Add the drops of spruce and lime, then plug in the diffuser and turn it on at the desired setting.

For additional consideration: Let the scent waft through you like an unexpected forest breeze, and feel your mind reach new heights.

BODY

Detoxification, Immune Boosting, Skin Tonics, Beauty Regimens and Digestive Aids

Your body is your temple — it's an old adage for good reason. Taking care of your physical well-being is a key component to a happy and healthy life. We all know that good diet and exercise, hygiene and regular sleep, and other good habits are the building blocks of physical wellness. But did you know that the power of aromatherapy can actually help your body in taking care of itself?

From the immune-boosting extracts of eucalyptus and myrrh, to the glandular-regulating properties of myrtle and lemongrass, the recipes in this section are designed to support your body's own healing and defense processes. There are also several recipes geared specifically towards the hair, skin, and other areas of beauty — the outward proof of true and holistic internal health. The cleansing essential oil of lemon and the purifying effects of peppermint are just a couple examples of how nature truly is the best cosmetics brand.

Pharmaceutical companies have built a billion-dollar industry by har-nessing the power of natural extracts to address all manner of physi-cal ailments. But with a cool-mist diffuser and these simple, effective recipes, you can become your own holistic healer — and just may be able to avoid having to make a trip to the pharmacy again!

BODY BLISS

---------------------★---------------------

They don't call strawflower the "everlasting daisy" for nothing. Enriching and supporting just about every system in the body at a cellular level, strawflower oil is prized for its rejuvenating properties and its seemingly miraculous ability to speed recovery from nagging illnesses or injury. This recipe also includes invigorating rosehip seed oil, which helps the body's tissue repair itself.

Ingredients:
★ 3 drops of strawflower oil
★ 3 drops of rosehip seed oil
★ 100 ml of water

Instructions: Fill the diffuser container with fresh water (straight from the tap, or distilled or filtered, depending on preference). Add the drops of strawflower and rosehip seed, then plug in the diffuser and turn it on at the desired setting.

For additional consideration: Your body will start to thank you just as soon as you inhale this light, lush blend. This is a wonderful recipe to use regularly in your diffuser anytime of year, but particularly in the autumn and winter months when we could all use a little extra nourishing.

JET-LAG BLASTER

Travel is wonderful – but the circadian disruptions caused by long distances and time changes are not so wonderful at all. This stabilizing blend of grapefruit, lime, and lavender is the perfect antidote to help get your body's rhythms back on track.

Ingredients:

★ 3 drops of grapefruit oil
★ 3 drops of lime oil
★ 3 drops of lavender oil
★ 100 ml of water

Instructions: Fill the diffuser container with fresh water (straight from the tap, or distilled or filtered, depending on preference). Add the drops of lavender, lime, and grapefruit, then plug in the diffuser and turn it on at the desired setting.

For additional consideration: This is the perfect blend to enjoy all the benefits of travel – while minimizing the downside. Take a few long inhales after your trip, and let your body take in the stabilizing power of this aromatic bouquet. And of course, have a wonderful trip!

HEADACHE HELP

There are few ailments worse than the common headache — and few mor
common. Next time you get that familiar pain in your head, try thi
relaxing and refreshing blend to help relieve tension and ease you
headache before reaching for the pill cabinet.

Ingredients:

★ 2 drops of marjoram oil

★ 2 drops of rosemary oil

★ 2 drops of lavender oil

★ 2 drops of thyme oil

★ 2 drops of peppermint oil

★ IOO ml of water

Instructions: Fill the diffuser container with fresh water (straigh
from the tap, or distilled or filtered, depending on preference). Ad
the drops of marjoram, thyme, rosemary, peppermint, lavender, then plu
in the diffuser and turn it on at the desired setting.

For additional consideration: Breathe in deeply and rub your temple
as you inhale this soothing blend. In no time at all, your headach
should start to ease, and a sense of calm should overcome your whol
body. Continue to rub your temples to compound the sense of relief, ar
feel better soon!

PURIFICATION CLEANSE

he combined cleansing powers of eucalyptus, lemon, and juniper berry
ils just can't be beat, and they come together in this powerful reci-
e designed to cleanse the body from the inside out. This is a particu-
arly useful blend to use during those long winter months when heat is
ore important than fresh air.

ngredients:

★ 3 drops of eucalyptus oil
★ 3 drops of lemon oil
★ 2 drops of juniper berry oil
★ IOO ml of water

nstructions: Fill the diffuser container with fresh water (straight
rom the tap, or distilled or filtered, depending on preference). Add
ie drops of eucalyptus, lemon, and juniper oil, then plug in the dif-
user and turn it on at the desired setting.

or additional consideration: It won't take long for this purifying
lend to cleanse and freshen the air around you, no matter how stuffy
ie space has become. Breathe deeply and enjoy the deep and clarifying
ffects of these bright, bracing aromas.

MIGRAINE HELPER

Migraines can be a serious downer – particularly when they strike in the midst of a busy day that won't allow you to just lay down in a darkened room until the pain subsides. For those unhappy times, this blend of lavender, lemongrass, and peppermint can be a godsend, helping you to feel better fast and get on with what needs to be done.

Ingredients:

★ 3 drops of lavender oil

★ 3 drops of lemongrass oil

★ 3 drops of peppermint oil

★ 100 ml of water

Instructions: Fill the diffuser container with fresh water (straight from the tap, or distilled or filtered, depending on preference). Add the drops of lavender, lemongrass, and peppermint oil, then plug in the diffuser and turn it on at the desired setting.

For additional consideration: This is a great blend to use when you need to keep moving despite your migraine. Breathe deeply and, with every exhale, visualize yourself expelling the pain of the migraine. Bit by bit, with every inhale of these soothing aromas, you should start to feel better and able to face the day.

WONDERFUL WELLNESS

This sweet and spicy aromatic blend is the perfect mix to put in your diffuser to promote overall health and well-being. Use this blend any time you want to give your body a pick-me-up, and enjoy the mix of fragrances that are sure to invigorate your whole system from the inside out.

Ingredients:

★ 2 drops of orange oil

★ 2 drops of cinnamon oil

★ 2 drops of rosemary oil

★ 2 drops of clove oil

★ 2 drops of eucalyptus oil

★ 100 ml of water

Instructions: Fill the diffuser container with fresh water (straight from the tap, or distilled or filtered, depending on preference). Add the drops of orange, clove, cinnamon, eucalyptus, and rosemary, then plug in the diffuser and turn it on at the desired setting.

For additional consideration: This is a great blend to use any time of day, any time of year, to support your system, cleanse your body, and to step up your overall health. Breathe deeply and smile, knowing you're doing your body good.

HERBACEOUS ENERGY BLEND

This wonderful mix of earthy aromas is designed to increase your energy levels and overall physiological vitality. The combination of basil, ginger and peppermint, with bracing frankincense and grounding rosemary, will empower your body from the inside out. Breathe deeply and enjoy!

Ingredients:
- ★ 2 drops of frankincense oil
- ★ 2 drops of basil oil
- ★ 2 drops of rosemary oil
- ★ 2 drops of ginger oil
- ★ 2 drops of peppermint oil
- ★ 100 ml of water

Instructions: Fill the diffuser container with fresh water (straight from the tap, or distilled or filtered, depending on preference). Add the drops of frankincense, ginger, basil, peppermint, and rosemary, then plug in the diffuser and turn it on at the desired setting.

For additional consideration: In no time at all this blend will have you feeling energized, stronger and more balanced. Enjoy the balanced power that this blend brings, and use it to seize the day!

LEMON CLEANSE

There is just nothing better than lemon for cleansing a body inside and out, and this simple ginger-citrus blend is the perfect mix for an easy, regular purification. Fill your space with these aromas anytime, day or night, and enjoy the open, healthy feeling of these compounds clearing out toxins and leaving freshness in their wake.

Ingredients:
★ 3 drops of lemon oil
★ 3 drops of ginger oil
★ 100 ml of water

Instructions: Fill the diffuser container with fresh water (straight from the tap, or distilled or filtered, depending on preference). Add the drops of lemon and ginger, then plug in the diffuser and turn it on at the desired setting.

For additional consideration: Breathe deeply and feel your airways and muscles become clearer and stronger with every inhale. This is a wonderful recipe to use around springtime to help alleviate the symptoms of seasonal allergies.

PURIFICATION POWER

Peppermint oil's purifying properties have been observed in laboratory studies, though aromatherapists have known for millennia that this sweet, invigorating compound is an excellent means of opening the lungs and cleansing the body. Mingled with soothing lavender and rosewood, this is a recipe to make you feel better if you're sick, and fantastic if you're well.

Ingredients:

★ 4 drops of peppermint oil

★ 2 drops of lavender oil

★ 2 drops of rosewood oil

★ 100 ml of water

Instructions: Fill the diffuser container with fresh water (straight from the tap, or distilled or filtered, depending on preference). Add the drops of rosewood, lavender, and peppermint, then plug in the diffuser and turn it on at the desired setting.

For additional consideration: Enjoy the refreshing power of this healing, purifying blend. Day or night, your body will feel cleaner and stronger, and your senses will thank you.

HEALING BREATH

Extract of the evergreen ravintsara tree is known for its health-giving properties around the world, and particularly its benefits to the respiratory system. This recipe blends the woody aroma of ravintsara oil with healing lavender and fresh citrus, perfect for soothing the body and opening the lungs.

Ingredients:

★ 4 drops of ravintsara oil

★ 2 drops of grapefruit oil

★ 100 ml of water

★ 2 drops of lemon oil

★ 1 drop of lavender oil

Instructions: Fill the diffuser container with fresh water (straight from the tap, or distilled or filtered, depending on preference). Add the drops of ravintsara, lemon, grapefruit, and lavender, then plug in the diffuser and turn it on at the desired setting.

For additional consideration: Take long, deep breaths, and let the restorative aromas heal your body. If you start feeling clearer and stronger after only a few inhales, don't worry - that means it's working!

RESPIRATORY RELIEF

Whether you're suffering from chest congestion, seasonal allergies, or any other respiratory ailment, this is a great blend to have in your diffuser. The combination of lemon, peppermint, eucalyptus, lime, rosemary and anise oils is the perfect way to clear your passage and breathe easier.

Ingredients:

★ 2 drops of lemon oil
★ 2 drops of eucalyptus oil
★ I drop of rosemary oil
★ I00 ml of water
★ 2 drops of peppermint oil
★ I drop of lime oil
★ I drop of anise oil

Instructions: Fill the diffuser container with fresh water (straight from the tap, or distilled or filtered, depending on preference). Add the drops of lemon, peppermint, eucalyptus, lime, rosemary, and anise, then plug in the diffuser and turn it on at the desired setting.

For additional consideration: Just a few deep breaths of these clarifying aromas, and you'll feel your respiratory system ease and work more freely. This is an excellent blend to help clear congestion and any other respiratory tract trouble, so use whenever you feel the need.

HANGOVER HELPER

Let's face it, some mornings your body is worse for wear — whether from alcohol, or too much work or play! This sweet blend is just what the aromatherapist ordered to help cleanse your body of toxins and restore the life to your cells. Laurel is a wonderful purifying agent, and is also known to support digestive function. With the clarifying zest of ginger and wild orange, this blend beats any hair of the dog.

Ingredients:

★ 4 drops of laurel oil
★ 2 drops of ginger oil
★ 2 drops of wild orange oil
★ 100 ml of water

Instructions: Fill the diffuser container with fresh water (straight from the tap, or distilled or filtered, depending on preference). Add the drops of laurel, ginger, and wild orange, then plug in the diffuser and turn it on at the desired setting.

For additional consideration: Relax and breathe deeply, and feel your mind and body start to heal. You'll be feeling better in no time — not to mention in love with these restorative fragrances.

PURIFYING STRENGTH

Clove is known for its powerful protective properties, and its extract is a wonderful ingredient for supporting overall immune strength. This wonderful blend adds the cleansing oil of grapefruit and plenty of healing lavender, for the ultimate recipe to cleanse and strengthen your body's essential natural defenses.

Ingredients:

★ 4 drops of clove oil

★ 2 drops of lavender oil

★ 1 drop of grapefruit oil

★ 100 ml of water

Instructions: Fill the diffuser container with fresh water (straight from the tap, or distilled or filtered, depending on preference). Add the drops of clove, lavender, and grapefruit, then plug in the diffuser and turn it on at the desired setting.

For additional consideration: This recipe is mellow enough to use in the evening before bedtime, though it also works great in the morning for sustained all-day strength.

CLEANSING RITUAL

This is a terrific blend for anytime your body needs holistic refreshment. Rejuvenating and purifying, the citrus and fennel blend is refreshing for home or office use. The grapefruit compounds are especially effective in helping to cleanse the body with every breath. For that reason, this is also an excellent recipe to use in conjunction with a weight-loss regime.

Ingredients:

★ 4 drops of grapefruit oil
★ 2 drops of tangerine oil
★ 2 drops of fennel oil
★ 100 ml of water

Instructions: Fill the diffuser container with fresh water (straight from the tap, or distilled or filtered, depending on preference). Add the drops of grapefruit, tangerine and fennel, then plug in the diffuser and turn it on at the desired setting.

For additional consideration: Enjoy this blend anytime of day or night, for a refreshing and cleansing atmosphere in every space. The fennel also makes this a good blend to promote digestive health.

CURB THOSE CRAVINGS

We all know what it takes to lead a healthy lifestyle — a balanced diet, and minimal intake of toxins such alcohol, nicotine, caffeine and junk foods. The hard part is reducing our powerful cravings for just such vices. This cleansing and energizing blend is the perfect support to help you resist temptations and make healthy choices.

Ingredients:

★ 3 drops of peppermint oil

★ 2 drops of spearmint oil

★ I drop of black pepper oil

★ 2 drops of bergamot oil

★ I drop of ylang-ylang oil

★ IOO ml of water

Instructions: Fill the diffuser container with fresh water (straight from the tap, or distilled or filtered, depending on preference). Add the drops of peppermint, bergamot, spearmint, ylang-ylang, and black pepper, then plug in the diffuser and turn it on at the desired setting.

For additional consideration: No matter what you're craving, a few long, deep breaths of this diffusion will help curb your appetite and replace it with a desire for something more healthy. So close your eyes, relax, and focus on your health — then take action to make it happen!

DELICIOUS DETOX

Who says that internal cleansing can't be luxurious too? The birch and sandalwood in this blend combine wonderfully for an earthy, clean scent, and work even better on the inside — cleansing out the organs and tissue and ridding the body of toxins. The touch of jasmine adds a taste of the exotic, and is itself an exceptionally effective sanitizing agent.

Ingredients:

★ 4 drops of birch oil
★ 3 drops of sandalwood oil
★ 2 drops of jasmine oil
★ 100 ml of water

Instructions: Fill the diffuser container with fresh water (straight from the tap, or distilled or filtered, depending on preference). Add the drops of birch, sandalwood, and jasmine, then plug in the diffuser and turn it on at the desired setting.

For additional consideration: Close your eyes for the first few breaths to fully appreciate this blend that's as delicious as it is beneficial.

CLEANSING CURE

This is an excellent blend to use any time your body is feeling weak or you suspect your immune system may be compromised. Whether you're in need of detoxification after a little too much partying, or you just want to give your system a refreshing cleanse, this is the blend for you.

Ingredients:

★ 3 drops of bergamot oil

★ 2 drops of lemon oil

★ 2 drops of juniper berry oil

★ 1 drop of fennel oil

★ 100 ml of water

Instructions: Fill the diffuser container with fresh water (straight from the tap, or distilled or filtered, depending on preference). Add the drops of bergamot, lemon, juniper berry, and fennel, then plug in the diffuser and turn it on at the desired setting.

For additional consideration: This delightfully fragrant blend will provide support to your entire system, supporting your immune factors and your internal organs, while calming a busy mind as an additional bonus.

CALMING CLEANSE

The combination of cypress, juniper, geranium, and lemon essential oils are a marvelous tonic for the entire body, and particularly the all-important lymphatic system. Use this blend any time you need to refresh your body from the inside out, and enjoy the clean, invigorating sensations that a few deep breaths will bring.

Ingredients:

★ 3 drops of cypress oil
★ 2 drops of juniper berry oil
★ 2 drops of lemon oil
★ 1 drop of geranium oil
★ 100 ml of water

Instructions: Fill the diffuser container with fresh water (straight from the tap, or distilled or filtered, depending on preference). Add the drops of cypress, juniper berry, lemon, and geranium, then plug in the diffuser and turn it on at the desired setting.

For additional consideration: This blend is an excellent restorative for the whole body. Breathe deeply and let the rich, earthy tones, balanced with floral and citrus notes, refresh your system and make you feel as calm and clean as if you were taking a spring stroll through the woods.

ANTI-EXHAUSTION

When life has got the better of you and you feel you're clean out of energy, try this energizing blend of peppermint, lavender and rosemary. This aromatic combination will help restore your internal power and regain the strength you need to get through the day — no matter how many tasks or challenges life has thrown your way.

Ingredients:

★ 4 drops of peppermint oil   ★ 2 drops of lavender oil

★ 2 drops of rosemary oil   ★ 100 ml of water

Instructions: Fill the diffuser container with fresh water (straight from the tap, or distilled or filtered, depending on preference). Add the drops of peppermint, lavender, and rosemary, then plug in the diffuser and turn it on at the desired setting.

For additional consideration: This is the blend to diffuse after you've just run a marathon — or if you simply feel that way. Take a few long inhales, and let this aromatic bouquet restore and revive your body in no time at all.

NASAL CLARITY

The extract of the myrtle plant's leaves and flower is a gentle, all-natural anti-inflammatory that works particularly well to clear respiratory passages. This blend combines the sanitizing myrtle oil with black pepper and jasmine, for a zesty fragrance that will have both your mind and your nasal cavities clean and clear in no time.

Ingredients:

★ 4 drops of myrtle oil
★ 2 drops of jasmine oil
★ I drop of black pepper oil
★ I00 ml of water

Instructions: Fill the diffuser container with fresh water (straight from the tap, or distilled or filtered, depending on preference). Add the drops of myrtle, jasmine, and black pepper, then plug in the diffuser and turn it on at the desired setting.

For additional consideration: You don't have to be feeling congested or clogged to benefit from this recipe. When you're healthy as a fiddle, the natural antiseptic properties of the myrtle oil keep your air fresh and clean — and help to keep your respiratory system in tip-top shape.

CALM AND CLEAN

This is a wonderful detoxifying recipe when your body needs to be energized as well as purified. Rich in refreshing citrus and the healing powers of chamomile, this recipe is a simple yet powerful blend to leave your body feeling rejuvenated and reinvigorated.

Ingredients:

★ 3 drops of lemon oil

★ 3 drops of chamomile

★ 1 drop of wild orange

★ 100 ml of water

Instructions: Fill the diffuser container with fresh water (straight from the tap, or distilled or filtered, depending on preference). Add the drops of lemon, chamomile, and wild orange, then plug in the diffuser and turn it on at the desired setting.

For additional consideration: Relax and prepare to feel refreshed all over. This diffused blend is a wonderful way to start the day, though thanks to the chamomile it's calming enough to use in the evenings.

HEALING POWER

The essence of pine is terrifically effective in treating a range of sinus infections, and even better in promoting sustained respiratory health. With notes of orange-blossom oil (also known as neroli) and cleansing grape-fruit, as well as healing lavender, this blend will fill your space with everything you need to breathe your best.

Ingredients:

★ 3 drops of pine oil

★ 2 drops of neroli oil

★ 2 drops of grapefruit oil

★ 100 ml of water

Instructions: Fill the diffuser container with fresh water (straight from the tap, or distilled or filtered, depending on preference). Add the drops of pine, neroli, and grapefruit oil, then plug in the diffuser and turn it on at the desired setting.

For additional consideration: Take in each breath knowing that your body is gaining strength and vitality. Don't be surprised if the world around you soon looks a little more inviting.

BREATHE FREE

This restorative floral blend is another excellent mix to support the sinuses and respiratory system. Nothing quite beats eucalyptus oil's power to cleanse the airways and refresh the lungs. With the soothing twin florals of lavender and geranium for extra healing power, this blend is perfect for when you want the most out of every breath.

Ingredients:

* ★ 3 drops of eucalyptus oil
* ★ 2 drops of lavender oil
* ★ 2 drops of geranium oil
* ★ 100 ml of water

Instructions: Fill the diffuser container with fresh water (straight from the tap, or distilled or filtered, depending on preference). Add the drops of eucalyptus, lavender, and geranium, then plug in the diffuser and turn it on at the desired setting.

For additional consideration: Feel your breath grow cleaner and stronger as you gently inhale and exhale these healing aromas. The geranium oil in this blend will also help balance out your body's hormones.

PURIFYING BREATH

This recipe is outstanding any time, but truly a godsend for those suffering from sinus or other respiratory trouble. The mix of menthol and coconut oil is an old home remedy going back centuries, and it's easy to understand why. This blend is both soothing and restorative, for mind as well as body.

Ingredients:

★ 5 drops of coconut oil
★ 3 drops of menthol oil
★ 100 ml of water

Instructions: Fill the diffuser container with fresh water (straight from the tap, or distilled or filtered, depending on preference). Add the drops of coconut and menthol, then plug in the diffuser and turn it on at the desired setting.

For additional consideration: Enjoy anytime of day or night, and refill as necessary — this blend does a lot of good, so get plenty of it!

HIBERNATE

Sometimes we all just need to shut out the world, be alone and still with ourselves, and hide from everything and everyone else for awhile. The soothing lavender in this blend, combined with cleansing lemon and healing spearmint, are perfect to help calm your senses and give your body the rejuvenating rest it needs.

Ingredients:

★ 5 drops of lavender oil

★ 2 drops of lemon oil

★ 1 drop of spearmint oil

★ 100 ml of water

Instructions: Fill the diffuser container with fresh water (straight from the tap, or distilled or filtered, depending on preference). Add the drops of lavender, lemon, and spearmint oils then plug in the diffuser and turn it on at the desired setting.

For additional consideration: This aromatic blend is likely to bring on a good, deep slumber. So let it. It will do you a world of good. When you wake up, you'll feel refreshed and ready to emerge from your hibernation.

IMMUNITY NOW

This is a terrific recipe to use around flu season, or anytime you're try-ing to ward off bugs or infections floating around the workplace or home. The eucalyptus oil and the ravintsara will work in tandem to both san-itize the air around you and support your body's own defenses, while the lavender is wonderful for healing and strengthening your respiratory and circulatory systems.

Ingredients:

★ 3 drops of eucalyptus oil
★ 3 drops of lavender oil
★ 2 drops of ravintsara oil
★ 100 ml of water

Instructions: Fill the diffuser container with fresh water (straight from the tap, or distilled or filtered, depending on preference). Add the drops of eucalyptus, lavender, and ravintsara, then plug in the diffuser and turn it on at the desired setting.

For additional consideration: As the diffuser mists out these health-giv-ing aromas, be sure to take time frequently for a few long, deep breaths - your body and your senses will thank you.

SELF-DEFENSE BLEND

There's no better feeling than a body that's strong and protected. This recipe packed with immunity-boosting extracts can help deliver that feeling, with the power of myrrh essential oils to activate and support our natural defense systems. The lemon and lavender add their restorative, healing properties to this disease-fighting blend.

Ingredients:

★ 4 drops of myrrh oil
★ 2 drops of lemon oil
★ 2 drops of lavender oil
★ 100 ml of water

Instructions: Fill the diffuser container with fresh water (straight from the tap, or distilled or filtered, depending on preference). Add the drops of myrrh, lemon, and lavender, then plug in the diffuser and turn it on at the desired setting.

For additional consideration: Every breath of this blend will help your body to protect itself from toxins and infections, so breathe deep and breathe easy. You're doing something great for yourself.

IMMUNITY BOOSTER

Here's another wonderful blend to use any time you want to support your immune system, perfect for strengthening your body's defenses in times of physical, emotional, or mental stress. Use when you're trying to ward off a cold, recover from illness, or just get by flu season unscathed.

Ingredients:

★ 2 drops of eucalyptus oil
★ I drop of rosemary oil
★ I drop of cinnamon oil
★ IOO ml of water

★ 2 drops of thyme oil
★ I drop of clove oil
★ I drop of orange oil

Instructions: Fill the diffuser container with fresh water (straight from the tap, or distilled or filtered, depending on preference). Add the drops of eucalyptus, thyme, rosemary, clove, cinnamon, and orange, then plug in the diffuser and turn it on at the desired setting.

For additional consideration: This blend is great to use any time you need a little extra strength, energizing and empowering you from the inside out. Whether you're recovering from sickness or just trying to prevent it, take several deep breaths and relax, knowing that you're doing your whole body a favor.

CRISP COOL-DOWN

When your body gets overheated, it can exhaust not only your physical system, but your mind and spirit as well. Use this refreshing blend to refresh your body, exhilarate your mind, and invigorate your spirit. This blend of peppermint and ylang-ylang feels a little like taking a long, cold drink of ice-water - a wonderful, cooling, cleansing favor for your whole body.

Ingredients:
★ 5 drops of peppermint oil
★ 3 drops of ylang-ylang oil
★ 100 ml of water

Instructions: Fill the diffuser container with fresh water (straight from the tap, or distilled or filtered, depending on preference). Add the drops of peppermint and ylang-ylang, then plug in the diffuser and turn it on at the desired setting.

For additional consideration: This is a great blend to use on a hot day, or after an exerting workout. Safely bringing down your body's temperature will help refresh your mind and spirit, giving you a feeling of coolness inside and out that is as calming as it is energizing.

IMMUNITY PLUS

Here's another power-house blend for the all-important immune system. Oregano and eucalyptus oils both are known to stimulate the body's defense systems, while the lavender and bergamot - among all their other benefits - aid in white-blood cell production.

Ingredients:

★ 3 drops of oregano oil

★ 2 drops of eucalyptus oil

★ 2 drops of lavender oil

★ 1 drop of bergamot oil

★ 100 ml of water

Instructions: Fill the diffuser container with fresh water (straight from the tap, or distilled or filtered, depending on preference). Add the drops of oregano, eucalyptus, lavender, and bergamot, then plug in the diffuser and turn it on at the desired setting.

For additional consideration: This diffusion blend is well balanced to use any time of the day or night, and is sure to leave you feeling stronger with a few deep breaths.

ENDOCRINE EXCELLENCE

Nurturing good endocrine function is one of the best ways to look out for your whole body. This terrific mix of detoxifying juniper berry, cooling cilantro and hormone-balancing rosemary is a wonderful recipe to use in sickness or health, sure to help support your body's natural equilibrium.

Ingredients:

★ 3 drops of cilantro oil

★ 2 drops of geranium oil

★ 100 ml of water

★ 2 drops of juniper berry oil

★ I drop of rosemary oil

Instructions: Fill the diffuser container with fresh water (straight from the tap, or distilled or filtered, depending on preference). Add the drops of cilantro, juniper berry, geranium, and rosemary, then plug in the diffuser and turn it on at the desired setting.

For additional consideration: This mix works well in the home or office, and is especially helpful around the holidays when stresses run high and the body's systems could use some extra help to stay steady and balanced.

ADRENAL AWESOME

A well-balanced adrenal system is essential to all your body's work, rest and play functions. Give it a balancing boost with this lovely blend of healing lavender, grounding basil, and the equilibrium-inducing extract of anise seed. You may feel fine now — but you're about to feel awesome.

Ingredients:
- ★ 4 drops of lavender
- ★ 2 drops of basil
- ★ 2 drop of anise seed
- ★ IOO ml of water

Instructions: Fill the diffuser container with fresh water (straight from the tap, or distilled or filtered, depending on preference). Add the drops of lavender, basil, and anise seed, then plug in the diffuser and turn it on at the desired setting.

For additional consideration: This blend is best to use in the morning, for the simple reason that you'll want the whole day to enjoy the stable, balanced energy it fosters. The anise seed has the added benefit of supporting digestive function, meaning this recipe is a great one to use if you're planning a large meal.

GLANDULAR GREATNESS

The extract of myrtle is well-known for its benefits to the respiratory system and to hair and skin health. But increasingly this essential oil is valued for its ability to stimulate the thyroid gland, which is important for everyone and particularly those who are trying to maintain a healthy body weight. The black licorice and lemongrass oils in this recipe have similar thyroid-supporting properties, and the licorice is even known to fight fatigue, depression, and other symptoms of imbalanced hormones.

Ingredients:

★ 4 drops of myrtle oil

★ 2 drops of lemongrass oil

★ 2 drops of black licorice oil

★ 100 ml of water

Instructions: Fill the diffuser container with fresh water (straight from the tap, or distilled or filtered, depending on preference). Add the drops of myrtle, black licorice, and lemongrass, then plug in the diffuser and turn it on at the desired setting.

For additional consideration: This blend gives a distinctive, herbaceous aroma, so it's perhaps best to keep this one for home use. You won't be sorry you did, once your body starts to enjoy the benefits of these amazing ingredients. Breathe deep and maximize your own internal balance.

CHILL OUT

If you're in need of a break, and a chance to calm down your system and give your body a rest, this is the blend for you. This crisp blend of grapefruit, orange, lemon, bergamot, and peppermint will have you feeling invigorated and rejuvenated.

Ingredients:

- ★ 2 drops of grapefruit oil
- ★ 2 drops of lemon oil
- ★ 2 drops of bergamot oil
- ★ 2 drops of orange oil
- ★ 2 drops of peppermint oil
- ★ 100 ml of water

Instructions: Fill the diffuser container with fresh water (straight from the tap, or distilled or filtered, depending on preference). Add the drops of grapefruit, orange, lemon, peppermint, and bergamot, then plug in the diffuser and turn it on at the desired setting.

For additional consideration: Breathe in deeply and take a good, deep dose of this cooling and refreshing blend. In no time at all, you will find yourself well and truly chilled out - and better off for it all over your body.

STOMACH STRENGTH

The digestive system is one of the most important and delicate in the body, and deserves extra special care for healthy upkeep. The rich antioxidants in carrot-seed oil and the toxin-eradicating properties in juniper berry extract, along with the grounding calm of a touch of bergamot, make this an excellent blend to keep your stomach strong and stable.

Ingredients:

★ 4 drops of carrot-seed oil   ★ 2 drops of juniper-berry oil

★ I drop of bergamot oil   ★ IOO ml of water

Instructions: Fill the diffuser container with fresh water (straight from the tap, or distilled or filtered, depending on preference). Add the drops of carrot seed, juniper berry, and bergamot, then plug in the diffuser and turn it on at the desired setting.

For additional consideration: A feeling of overall physical calm should come fast after several long, deep breaths of this cool-mist blend. This is a great recipe to use before, during, or after a large meal, to support optimally comfortable digestion.

PMS-BE-GONE

When you know that you've got your time of the month coming up — and the cramps, bloating, and muscle aches to confirm it — this is the best blend to have in your diffuser. The clary sage, ylang-ylang, lavender, and peppermint oils in this blend are the perfect way to calm your internal system and regulate your hormones, easing the symptoms of premenstrual syndrome for even the most extreme cases.

Ingredients:
- ★ 3 drops of clary sage
- ★ 2 drops of ylang-ylang oil
- ★ 2 drops of lavender oil
- ★ 2 drops of peppermint oil
- ★ 100 ml of water

Instructions: Fill the diffuser container with fresh water (straight from the tap, or distilled or filtered, depending on preference). Add the drops of clary sage, ylang-ylang, lavender, and peppermint, then plug in the diffuser and turn it on at the desired setting.

For additional consideration: Take in several deep inhales of this soothing blend, and enjoy the sensation of these aromas as they balance the hormones, relax the muscles, and alleviate the premenstrual symptoms you may be experiencing.

TIME OF THE MONTH

Menstruating ladies, this blend's for you. The soothing and mildly analgesic properties of the clary sage oil are perfectly complemented by uplifting lemongrass and hormone-balancing geranium. No one said this time of the month has to be miserable - with this aromatic mix in your diffuser, your body's tensions will start to ease soon enough.

Ingredients:

★ 2 drops of clary sage oil

★ 2 drops of geranium oil

★ 2 drops of lemongrass oil

★ 100 ml of water

Instructions: Fill the diffuser container with fresh water (straight from the tap, or distilled or filtered, depending on preference). Add the drops of clary sage, lemongrass, and geranium, then plug in the diffuser and turn it on at the desired setting.

For additional consideration: This recipe's ratios can be adjusted according to individual needs. In particular, those experiencing especially intense cramps might want to add an extra drop or two of that wonderful clary sage, for faster relief.

MORNING SICKNESS RELIEVER

Pregnancy is a miraculous and magical time in a woman's life, and a blessing for the whole family. Unfortunately, the first trimester of that miraculous magical blessing can come with some pretty nauseating side-effects - chiefly, morning sickness. This blend is a great all-natural way to alleviate it, though it's best to limit the diffusing time to 10-15 minutes maximum due to increased sensitivity to smells during pregnancy. If ever in doubt, pregnant women should check with their doctors to ensure safe aromatherapy diffusion.

Ingredients:

★ 4 drops of spearmint oil   ★ 2 drops of ginger oil
★ 1 drop of lime oil   ★ 100 ml of water

Instructions: Fill the diffuser container with fresh water (straight from the tap, or distilled or filtered, depending on preference). Add the drops of spearmint, ginger, and lime, then plug in the diffuser and turn it on at the desired setting.

For additional consideration: If chronic morning sickness has marred your first trimester, diffuse this blend regularly to help ease the affliction and provide much needed relief. Breathe deeply and enjoy your pregnancy - and get ready for the bundle of joy to come!

LABOR PAINS

While childbirth is a natural process, there is a very good reason they call it "labor" — it can be hard work! To help keep you relaxed and calm, and to ease yourself through those painful contractions, diffuse this blend once labor has commenced.

Ingredients:

★ 3 drops of lavender oil
★ I drop of ylang-ylang oil
★ I drop of clary sage oil
★ 2 drops of frankincense oil
★ I drop of chamomile oil
★ IOO ml of water

Instructions: Fill the diffuser container with fresh water (straight from the tap, or distilled or filtered, depending on preference). Add the drops of lavender, frankincense, ylang-ylang, chamomile, and clary sage, then plug in the diffuser and turn it on at the desired setting.

For additional consideration: This is a great blend to have in your diffuser, whether you're giving birth in a hospital room or at home. I can't pretend that it will make labor easy or painless — but it sure will help. Breathe deeply, and prepare to deliver your bundle of joy.

ALLERGY RELIEF

This blend is an excellent all-natural alternative to drugs and chemicals to help alleviate the symptoms of allergic rhinitis, also known as hay fever, along with other non life-threatening allergies. The combination of lavender, lemon, and peppermint are the perfect way to calm your immune system and breathe easier in no time.

Ingredients:

★ 3 drops of lavender oil
★ 3 drops of lemon oil
★ 3 drops of peppermint oil
★ 100 ml of water

Instructions: Fill the diffuser container with fresh water (straight from the tap, or distilled or filtered, depending on preference). Add the drops of lavender, lemon, and peppermint, then plug in the diffuser and turn it on at the desired setting.

For additional consideration: With a few deep breaths, you'll feel your immune system starting to calm and your breathing come easier. Allergies are no way to go through life, so take several long inhales and enjoy feeling better fast — and then getting on with a great day!

COLD AND FLU BUSTER

As the name suggests, this is the perfect blend for warding off colds or the flu. Even if you don't feel sickness coming on, the lemon, thyme, eucalyptus, and peppermint are the perfect combination to cleanse the air and keep yourself feeling healthy and your body clean and strong.

Ingredients:

★ 3 drops of peppermint oil

★ 2 drops of thyme oil

★ 100 ml of water

★ 3 drops of eucalyptus oil

★ 1 drop of lemon oil

Instructions: Fill the diffuser container with fresh water (straight from the tap, or distilled or filtered, depending on preference). Add the drops of peppermint, eucalyptus, thyme, and lemon, then plug in the diffuser and turn it on at the desired setting.

For additional consideration: This is the ideal blend to diffuse when you need that internal pick-me-up for your whole system. Even if it's not winter, we can all be prone to the winter blues - and this blend is the perfect way to chase them away and make you feel like spring is in the air.

DECONGESTANT

There's nothing worse than having a cold or the flu and suffering from the stuffed-up nose that comes along with it. This powerful, cleansing blend of eucalyptus, thyme, and lime is the perfect way to clear your passages and breathe a little easier.

Ingredients:

★ 2 drops of eucalyptus oil

★ 2 drops of thyme oil

★ 1 drop of lime oil

★ 100 ml of water

Instructions: Fill the diffuser container with fresh water (straight from the tap, or distilled or filtered, depending on preference). Add the drops of eucalyptus, thyme, and lime, then plug in the diffuser and turn it on at the desired setting.

For additional consideration: This powerful decongestant is gentle enough to use even when you're feeling your worst and when your immune system is at its lowest. A few deep breaths, and you'll be feeling better in no time – what a difference a clearer respiratory system can make!

DIGESTIVE CALM

This mix will be a welcome aromatic addition to any space, but especially so for those whose stomachs may need a little settling. The incomparable mix of grounding bergamot, soothing patchouli, and healing digestion-friendly fennel is a balm to the troubled gut.

Ingredients:

★ 4 drops of fennel oil
★ 2 drops of bergamot oil
★ 2 drops of patchouli oil
★ 100 ml of water

Instructions: Fill the diffuser container with fresh water (straight from the tap, or distilled or filtered, depending on preference). Add the drops of fennel, bergamot, and patchouli, then plug in the diffuser and turn it on at the desired setting.

For additional consideration: Sit back and enjoy, and know that you're doing your entire digestive system a healthy favor. Use this recipe in your diffuser day or night, perhaps with the addition of a hot water bottle for those with tummy-ache.

CHAI LATTE

I'm a huge tea lover and chai lattes are my particular weakness. There's nothing I love better than a hot cup of chai latte after a big meal — which can be a problem if that meal happens to fall a few hours before bedtime. This blend of cardamom, cinnamon, ginger and clove is the perfect substitute — an aromatic equivalent to my beloved chai lattes, with none of the caffeine to keep me awake!

Ingredients:

★ 2 drops of cardamom oil

★ 2 drops of cinnamon oil

★ 2 drops of clove oil

★ 2 drops of ginger oil

★ 100 ml of water

Instructions: Fill the diffuser container with fresh water (straight from the tap, or distilled or filtered, depending on preference). Add the drops of cardamom, cinnamon, clove, and ginger, then plug in the diffuser and turn it on at the desired setting.

For additional consideration: This warming blend will help soothe the stomach and settle the senses. Use it any time you're craving a cup of tea — but don't actually want to drink the caffeine. Instead, breathe in these wonderful aromas and enjoy all the benefits of a good chai latte, with none of the downsides.

BELLY BALM

Here's another wonderful recipe to soothe the stomach and support overall intestinal health. This sweet and soothing mix combines the digestive-healing powers of fennel oil with the restorative essences of lavender and rose.

Ingredients:

★ 4 drops of fennel oil

★ 2 drops of lavender oil

★ 2 drops of rose oil

★ 100 ml of water

Instructions: Fill the diffuser container with fresh water (straight from the tap, or distilled or filtered, depending on preference). Add the drops of fennel, lavender, and rose, then plug in the diffuser and turn it on at the desired setting.

For additional consideration: Breathe deep and relax, letting these feel-good fragrances take care of the rest. This recipe is an excellent choice to drop into your diffuser after a large meal, or any time you want to help your body process with ease.

ALL-DAY STRONG

The rosemary in this blend is a wonderful way to stimulate and refresh your whole system. Rosemary tends to have a clarifying effect on the respiratory system, which provides extra energy to all your cells throughout the day. Peppermint and lemon are the perfect complement, for a grounding, strengthening aromatic bouquet.

Ingredients:

★ 4 drops of rosemary oil

★ 3 drops of peppermint oil

★ 2 drops of lemon oil

★ 100 ml of water

Instructions: Fill the diffuser container with fresh water (straight from the tap, or distilled or filtered, depending on preference). Add the drops of rosemary, peppermint, and lemon, then plug in the diffuser and turn it on at the desired setting.

For additional consideration: Whether it's getting towards the end of a long day, or if you're only just getting started, this is a brightening blend that will give your body the boost it needs to power through and feel great.

WORKOUT WONDERFUL

This terrific blend of peppermint, orange, and grapefruit essential oils is a terrific tonic for your whole body, lending energy, stamina and strength to your system. Use this blend before or during workouts to add power to your exercise routine, and keep you strong and focused throughout.

Ingredients:
★ 3 drops of peppermint oil
★ 2 drops of grapefruit oil
★ 3 drops of orange oil
★ 100 ml of water

Instructions: Fill the diffuser container with fresh water (straight from the tap, or distilled or filtered, depending on preference). Add the drops of peppermint, orange, and grapefruit, then plug in the diffuser and turn it on at the desired setting.

For additional consideration: Whether you're diffusing this blend at the start of your workout to get you pumped up, or using it throughout to keep you going, these aromas are the perfect way to see your body through to keep fit and strong. Breathe deeply, and feel wonderful throughout your workout!

3 P.M. REVIVAL

Instead of reaching for a chocolate bar to see you through the end of a long day, try diffusing this revitalizing blend instead. This wonderful mix of peppermint, orange, and rosemary will revive those flagging energy levels and help you focus on what needs to be done.

Ingredients:

★ 3 drops of peppermint oil
★ 3 drops of orange oil
★ 2 drops of rosemary oil
★ 100 ml of water

Instructions: Fill the diffuser container with fresh water (straight from the tap, or distilled or filtered, depending on preference). Add the drops of peppermint, orange, and rosemary, then plug in the diffuser and turn it on at the desired setting.

For additional consideration: This is a terrific blend to ward off the mid-afternoon blahs. The energizing aromas are mellow enough to use through the early evening, with no risk of making it difficult to sleep at night. A few deep breaths of this blend, and you'll feel refreshed and ready to finish the day strong!

STRONG AND STABLE

This is a refreshing "anytime" blend to support your body's energy levels and physical sense of well-being. Both thyme and tea-tree oil are excellent system stabilizers, while the geranium extract helps to heal the damage of built-up stress and toxins in the body. All three extracts also work as powerful immune-system support.

Ingredients:

★ 3 drops of thyme oil

★ 3 drops of tea-tree oil

★ 3 drops of geranium oil

★ 100 ml of water

Instructions: Fill the diffuser container with fresh water (straight from the tap, or distilled or filtered, depending on preference). Add the drops of thyme, tea tree, and geranium, then plug in the diffuser and turn it on at the desired setting.

For additional consideration: Take a few deep inhales, close your eyes, and see if you can't feel your cells whispering a happy "thank you" for this enriching diffusion. This recipe is a well-balanced addition to a holistic lifestyle.

BEAUTY MIST

This simple but powerful blend has been used for millennia by women seeking a clean, healthy glow to their skin. Rosehip oil is tremendously rich in the essential fatty acids that keep skin radiant and fresh, while the lavender soothes and tones the pores to leave you silky and smooth.

Ingredients:

★ 4 drops of rosehip oil

★ 3 drops of lavender oil

★ 100 ml of water

Instructions: Fill the diffuser container with fresh water (straight from the tap, or distilled or filtered, depending on preference). Add the drops of rosehip and lavender, then plug in the diffuser and turn it on at the desired setting.

For additional consideration: This blend is ideal for continuous use throughout the day, so don't be afraid to go for successive diffusions. It only takes a few long, deep breaths, however, for your skin to start feeling youthful and looking beautiful. Enjoy!

PORE CLEANSE

The best part of a professional salon facial is the pore-cleansing mist at the beginning. This diffuser recipe brings all those pore-cleansing benefits without the humidifier and without those salon prices. The extract of oak moss in this blend is an extraordinarily effective detoxifier that works wonders on the skin, and combines with the lavender and geranium for full-body purification and relaxation.

Ingredients:

★ 4 drops of oak moss oil
★ I drop of geranium oil

★ 2 drops of lavender oil
★ I00 ml of water

Instructions: Fill the diffuser container with fresh water (straight from the tap, or distilled or filtered, depending on preference). Add the drops of oak moss, lavender, and geranium, then plug in the diffuser and turn it on at the desired setting.

For additional consideration: This recipe is most effective on clean skin, so it's a great one to use in your diffuser after a bath or shower. It's best to wait until the diffusion has run out to apply any skin moisturizers, as that will help lock in the benefits of the essential oils for your pores.

SKIN SAVER

This clove and coconut-rich blend is ideal for preventing acne break-outs, as well as for general skin health and cleansing. The touch of wild orange adds a refreshing citrus zest, which will help rejuvenate the entire body and tighten up pores. This recipe is best for morning use, providing a healing and protective treatment whose benefits will last throughout the day.

Ingredients:

★ 3 drops of clove oil

★ 2 drops of wild orange oil

★ 3 drops of coconut oil

★ 100 ml of water

Instructions: Fill the diffuser container with fresh water (straight from the tap, or distilled or filtered, depending on preference). Add the drops of clove, coconut, and wild orange, then plug in the diffuser and turn it on at the desired setting.

For additional consideration: With an efficient cool-mist diffuser, there's no need to stay close to the source to get the full benefits of the blend on your skin and pores — just breathe in, smile, and know that you're making your skin very happy.

COSMETIC CURE

You know those times when you've worn too much makeup, drank too much alcohol, or gotten too much sun – those days when your skin is just begging for a break? If so, this is the recipe for you. The rejuvenating, lipid-supporting properties of tangerine, coconut and avocado cannot be underestimated to refresh and replenish the skin's essential nutrients.

Ingredients:

★ 5 drops of avocado oil

★ 2 drops of tangerine oil

★ 1 drop of coconut oil

★ 100 ml of water

Instructions: Fill the diffuser container with fresh water (straight from the tap, or distilled or filtered, depending on preference). Add the drops of avocado, tangerine, and coconut oil, then plug in the diffuser and turn it on at the desired setting.

For additional consideration: This is a wonderful recipe for day or night, though particularly effective in the morning when your skin will best absorb the healing properties.

AROMATIC FACIAL

The amazing carrot-seed extract proves its value once again, with its wonderful antioxidant properties at work in this anti-aging skincare blend. The mild, sweet carrot-seed fragrance is balanced by soothing lavender and cleansing lime, to leave your skin as happy as your senses.

Ingredients:

★ 4 drops of carrot-seed oil

★ 4 drops of lavender oil

★ 2 drops of lime

★ 100 ml of water

Instructions: Fill the diffuser container with fresh water (straight from the tap, or distilled or filtered, depending on preference). Add the drops of carrot-seed, lavender, and lime, then plug in the diffuser and turn it on at the desired setting.

For additional consideration: The calming effects of the lavender make this a particularly good blend to use in the afternoon or evenings. Don't worry – if you do wind up falling into a relaxed sleep, you can rest easy knowing that your skin is getting its very own spa treatment.

SUPER SKIN

The cajuput essential oil in this recipe is an outstanding all-around cleanser, detoxifier and antiseptic, and has long been used to help prevent and heal acne. This blend includes extract of angelica — a serene aroma and general calmant known in Germany as the "oil of angels" — and soothing lavender to help skin feel and look its freshest.

Ingredients:

★ 3 drops of cajuput oil
★ 3 drops of lavender oil
★ 3 drops of angelica oil
★ 100 ml of water

Instructions: Fill the diffuser container with fresh water (straight from the tap, or distilled or filtered, depending on preference). Add the drops of cajuput, lavender, and angelica, then plug in the diffuser and turn it on at the desired setting.

For additional consideration: Enjoy this beautifying blend anytime your skin could use some purification — this is an especially good recipe for those with oily skin. Afterwards, splash your face with cold water for a final rinse that will help your pores lock in the benefits of the treatment.

SCENTED SCAR VANISHER

This deceptively simple blend makes excellent use of the unique properties of lavandin oil, the extract from a hybrid plant known for its unmatched support in treating wounds of all kinds. Like the hyssop oil it's mixed with here, lavandin acts as both an antiseptic to protect minor cuts from infection, and as an agent of cell repair that will help erase unsightly scars and other skin blemishes.

Ingredients:

★ 3 drops of lavandin oil   ★ 3 drops of hyssop oil

★ IOO ml of water

Instructions: Fill the diffuser container with fresh water (straight from the tap, or distilled or filtered, depending on preference). Add the drops of lavandin and hyssop, then plug in the diffuser and turn it on at the desired setting.

For additional consideration: Don't be afraid to add an extra drop or two of either essential oil in this recipe. These aromas are nothing but beneficial, not just for the skin but for the whole body, so sit back and take in the healing cool mist.

HAIR HEAVEN

You don't need to shampoo your hair to enjoy all the enriching benefits that essential oils can bring to your scalp and locks. For support growing a lustrous head of hair - or simply for a wonderful smelling, cleansing, and antioxidant-rich aromatic space - try this blend of peppermint, rosemary, lemon and basil in your diffuser.

Ingredients:

* ★ 4 drops of peppermint oil
* ★ 2 drops of rosemary oil
* ★ 2 drops of lemon oil
* ★ 1 drop of basil oil
* ★ 100 ml of water

Instructions: Fill the diffuser container with fresh water (straight from the tap, or distilled or filtered, depending on preference). Add the drops of peppermint, rosemary, lemon and basil, then plug in the diffuser and turn it on at the desired setting.

For additional consideration: This blend is great because it can benefit any type of hair. The peppermint and lemon are cleansing and stimulate the scalp to aid hair growth, while the basil's and rosemary's restorative properties are great for strengthening follicle roots and giving hair a silky sheen.

HEALING BEAUTY

Whoever said "beauty hurts" was flat out wrong – or at least they never enjoyed this luscious mixture of soothing lavender, clarifying rose, and rejuvenating strawflower oil (better known to hair and skin experts as "immortelle" or the "everlasting daisy"). This blend give your pores deep restorative treatment and leaves you looking great and feeling even better.

Ingredients:

★ 4 drops of strawflower oil
★ 2 drops of rose oil

★ 2 drops of lavender oil
★ 100 ml of water

Instructions: Fill the diffuser container with fresh water (straight from the tap, or distilled or filtered, depending on preference). Add the drops of strawflower, lavender, and rose oil, then plug in the diffuser and turn it on at the desired setting.

For additional consideration: The lavender and strawflower oils will start stimulating cell repair right from the first inhale. It will only take a couple of more breaths before the rose extract kicks in to lend a clean, flushed glow to the cheeks.

AROMATIC MUSCLE MASSAGE

This blend helps your body restore and relax, both excellent for alle-viating muscle tension and building healthy tissue. Clarity sage is a wonderful all body calming agent and natural pain reliever, and works perfectly with sandalwood and wild orange in this blend to shed stress, relax the muscles and rejuvenate your system at a cellular level.

Ingredients:

★ 4 drops of clarity sage oil
★ 2 drops of wild orange oil
★ 2 drops of sandalwood oil
★ 100 ml of water

Instructions: Fill the diffuser container with fresh water (straight from the tap, or distilled or filtered, depending on preference). Add the drops of clary sage, sandalwood, and wild orange, then plug in the diffuser and turn it on at the desired setting.

For additional consideration: This blend is perfect after a rigorous workout or simply to keep your body loose and happy during a tough day. It's not likely to make you sleepy, so it's fine for morning time just be prepared for the ultimate muscle massage *without* the massage.

SWEET RELIEF

The extract of the hyssop plant's purple flowers are a wonderful support to the circulatory system, and for that reason is often used to alleviate rheumatism and other forms of joint pain. This lovely blend adds soothing touches of melissa oil and sweet, detoxifying tangerine.

Ingredients:

★ 4 drops of hyssop oil

★ 2 drops of tangerine oil

★ 2 drops of melissa oil

★ 100 ml of water

Instructions: Fill the diffuser container with fresh water (straight from the tap, or distilled or filtered, depending on preference). Add the drops of hyssop, melissa, and tangerine, then plug in the diffuser and turn it on at the desired setting.

For additional consideration: This mild, mellowing blend is refreshing enough to use during the day without getting tired, and exceptionally helpful in the evenings when sore joints might be flaring up. Take a moment to close your eyes and inhale deeply, savoring the sweet relief of this health giving blend.

LIGHTEN AND LIFT

The combined uplifting powers of bergamot, lavender, and geranium are certain to brighten the atmosphere and lift moods in any space. This powerful, energizing blend is perfect to diffuse at a gathering to create a cheerful vibe, or when you're alone and trying to brighten your own spirits.

Ingredients:
★ 3 drops of bergamot oil
★ 3 drops of lavender oil
★ 2 drops of geranium oil
★ 100 ml of water

Instructions: Fill the diffuser container with fresh water (straight from the tap, or distilled or filtered, depending on preference). Add the drops of bergamot, lavender, and geranium, then plug in the diffuser and turn it on at the desired setting.

For additional consideration: This uplifting and refreshing blend is a wonderful way to cheer up any space. Breathe deeply and feel your spirits lift with every inhale...and enjoy!

WINTER CELEBRATION

The uplifting and sweetly spiced aromas in this rich blend is the perfect way to add a little warmth and cheer to any winter gathering. The patchouli and ylang-ylang will help lift everyone's mood, while the cinnamon, orange, clove and white fir create a delicious aromatic bouquet to help everyone feel that much more merry!

Ingredients:

★ 3 drops of patchouli oil

★ 1 drop of orange oil

★ 1 drop of ylang-ylang oil

★ 100 ml of water

★ 2 drops of cinnamon oil

★ 1 drop of clove oil

★ 1 drop of white fir oil

Instructions: Fill the diffuser container with fresh water (straight from the tap, or distilled or filtered, depending on preference). Add the drops of patchouli, cinnamon, orange, clove, ylang-ylang, and white fir, then plug in the diffuser and turn it on at the desired setting.

For additional consideration: This spicy blend will have your heart and home warm and cheery in no time. The weather outside may be frightful, but in a few short minutes, these aromas will have your space feeling purely delightful!

ZENERGIZE

This recipe is both uplifting and relaxing, designed to stimulate the senses and optimize the body's internal systems. This blend of invigorating spruce and rosewood, is combined with the refreshing coconut and healing powers of frankincense.

Ingredients:

★ 3 drops of spruce oil
★ 3 drops of coconut oil
★ I drop of frankincense
★ I drop of rosewood
★ IOO ml of water

Instructions: Fill the diffuser container with fresh water (straight from the tap, or distilled or filtered, depending on preference). Add the drops of spruce, coconut, frankincense, and rosewood, then plug in the diffuser and turn it on at the desired setting.

For additional consideration: Enjoy the feeling of your entire body getting the rejuvenating air it craves. This recipe is perfect to use before or during a good workout, or anytime your body needs a dose of sustained, healthful energy.

WALK IN THE WOODS

There's nothing quite like a long walk in the woods on a crisp morning to clear your mind and lift your spirits. But if you, like me, don't live anywhere near the woods and don't have the time on most mornings for a long walk of any location, this wonderful woody blend is a very close second to get that same refreshed, positive feeling!

Ingredients:

★ 3 drops of sandalwood oil
★ I drop of frankincense oil
★ IOO ml of water
★ 2 drops of spearmint oil
★ I drop of juniper berry oil

Instructions: Fill the diffuser container with fresh water (straight from the tap, or distilled or filtered, depending on preference). Add the drops of sandalwood, spearmint, frankincense, and juniper berry, then plug in the diffuser and turn it on at the desired setting.

For additional consideration: These herbaceous and crisp aromas combine to create the perfect mix that will soon take you away from your stresses, and help you reconnect with what's important. Breathe deeply and let yourself be transported to that wonderful mood that a walk in the woods can bring...even if you're nowhere near the forest!

FRESH AND FIT

Grapefruit is one of the best ingredients around for those looking to control their weight or shed a few pounds. That's because it's both a natural detoxifier, and a mild appetite suppressant. Both properties are enhanced in this energizing blend of ylang-ylang oil, palmarosa extract and ginger.

Ingredients:

★ 4 drops of grapefruit oil

★ 2 drops of ginger oil

★ 100 ml of water

★ 2 drops of palmarosa oil

★ 1 drop of ylang-ylang oil

Instructions: Fill the diffuser container with fresh water (straight from the tap, or distilled or filtered, depending on preference). Add the drops of grapefruit, palmarosa, ginger, and ylang-ylang, then plug in the diffuser and turn it on at the desired setting.

For additional consideration: This uplifting and refreshing blend is a wonderful way to cheer up any space. Breathe deeply and feel your spirits lift with every inhale. This recipe is a great way to enhance the benefits of a healthy diet and active lifestyle. While the grapefruit and ginger cleanse the body and curb the impulse to overeat, the ylang-ylang and palmarosa will keep you calm and energized to support proper metabolic function. Breathe deeply and enjoy!

WEIGHT LOSS WONDER

Here's another recipe that packs the power of grapefruit extract to support a lean diet and promote detoxification. It's blended here with the soothing, protective clove oil for an overall immunity boost, and a healthy dose of fennel to nurture the digestive system.

Ingredients:

★ 4 drops of grapefruit oil

★ 3 drops of fennel oil

★ 1 drop of clove oil

★ 100 ml of water

Instructions: Fill the diffuser container with fresh water (straight from the tap, or distilled or filtered, depending on preference). Add the drops of grapefruit, fennel, and clove, then plug in the diffuser and turn it on at the desired setting.

For additional consideration: This is one of those great "anytime" blends that works morning or night. You might find it especially welcome at the beginning of the day, with these crisp, restorative fragrances working together to start your system off right. With healthy foods and regular exercise along with this aromatic mix, shedding a few pounds has never been so delicious!

SWEET SLEEP

A good night's sleep is absolutely crucial for overall health and well being. This recipe is perfect for those times when your body needs a little extra encouragement to shut down. The lavender and roman chamomile support restfulness throughout the body and mind, and the thyme in this blend is additionally known for promoting deep sleep and warding off nightmares.

Ingredients:
★ 3 drops of lavender oil
★ 3 drops of roman chamomile oil
★ 2 drops of thyme oil
★ 100 ml of water

Instructions: Fill the diffuser container with fresh water (straight from the tap, or distilled or filtered, depending on preference). Add the drops of lavender, roman chamomile, thyme, then plug in the diffuser and turn it on at the desired setting.

For additional consideration: Settle into bed for a restful night. This recipe should help to stimulate calming and soothing thoughts, perfect to drift off into a deep and restorative sleep. Avoid this recipe in the mornings or during the day.

SUMMER NIGHT

This wonderful blend of citronella, peppermint, spearmint and lemongrass is a cooling mix that will freshen your body and invigorate your system. Bonus? It's a fantastic mosquito repellant, making it the perfect blend to use on any hot summer night.

Ingredients:

★ 4 drops of citronella oil
★ 2 drops of peppermint oil
★ I drop of spearmint oil
★ I drop of lemongrass oil
★ IOO ml of water

Instructions: Fill the diffuser container with fresh water (straight from the tap, or distilled or filtered, depending on preference). Add the drops of citronella, peppermint, spearmint, and lemongrass, then plug in the diffuser and turn it on at the desired setting.

For additional consideration: This cooling blend is like a fresh breeze — making it perfect for a balmy summer's night, minus the mosquitoes! Breathe deeply and enjoy the fresh, happy scent of summer.

ALL-NATURAL INSECT REPELLANT

Creepy crawlies have always been irritants, and vectors of disease and other health hazards. With the onset of the zika virus now being carried by mosquitoes, it's more important than ever to use every tool available to try to keep the bugs away. This blend of lemongrass, tea tree, thyme, eucalyptus, and rosemary oils is a great place to start.

Ingredients:

★ 2 drops of lemongrass oil

★ 2 drops of tea tree oil

★ 2 drop of thyme oil

★ 2 drop of eucalyptus oil

★ 1 drop of rosemary oil

★ 100 ml of water

Instructions: Fill the diffuser container with fresh water (straight from the tap, or distilled or filtered, depending on preference). Add the drops of lemongrass, tea tree, thyme, eucalyptus, and rosemary oil, then plug in the diffuser and turn it on at the desired setting.

For additional consideration: Use this blend any time you want to prevent those creepy crawlies from crashing your party. This blend will banish them in no time, ensuring that everyone can relax and enjoy themselves in safety and health.

SPRING CLEANING

Nothing cleanses the air quite like citrus, making this lemon, orange, lime, and grapefruit combination a powerful diffusion to freshen the air. This is the perfect blend to diffuse to put a spring in your step while you're getting your house in order - clean mind, clean body, clean atmosphere means optimal health!

Ingredients:

* ★ 3 drops of orange oil
* ★ 2 drops of lime oil
* ★ 100 ml of water
* ★ 2 drops of lemon oil
* ★ 2 drop of grapefruit oil

Instructions: Fill the diffuser container with fresh water (straight from the tap, or distilled or filtered, depending on preference). Add the drops of orange, lemon, lime, and grapefruit, then plug in the diffuser and turn it on at the desired setting.

For additional consideration: This blend will have your air feeling cleaner and fresher in no time at all - and help you stay balanced and focused as you go about your cleaning and other household chores. There's no reason to dread spring cleaning with this aromatic bouquet in your diffuser, so breathe deeply and enjoy tidying up!

FIRST DATE

There's nothing quite so exciting as a first rendezvous with a potential love interest — and nothing more anxiety-inducing! This blend of grounding bergamot, uplifting ylang-ylang, and calming frankincense is the perfect aromatic combination to use before or during a first date as the antidote to those nerves and jitters – and have a great time.

Ingredients:
★ 4 drops of bergamot oil
★ 2 drops of ylang-ylang oil
★ I drop of frankincense oil
★ IOO ml of water

Instructions: Fill the diffuser container with fresh water (straight from the tap, or distilled or filtered, depending on preference). Add the drops of bergamot, ylang-ylang, and frankincense, then plug in the diffuser and turn it on at the desired setting.

For additional consideration: With a few deep breaths of this diffusion, you'll find your nerves ebbing and the conversation flowing — along with, just maybe...a little romance!

AROMA ROMANCE

The combination of zinging black pepper, uplifting grapefruit, and sensual jasmine creates the perfect aromatic blend to stimulate a romantic atmosphere and intimate emotional exchange.

Ingredients:

★ 3 drops of black pepper oil
★ 3 drops of grapefruit oil
★ 3 drops of jasmine oil
★ 100 ml of water

Instructions: Fill the diffuser container with fresh water (straight from the tap, or distilled or filtered, depending on preference). Add the drops of black pepper, grapefruit, and jasmine, then plug in the diffuser and turn it on at the desired setting.

For additional consideration: Whether you're using this diffusion on a first date or on a fifty first, this delicious blend will create a perfect setting for romantic connection. Breathe deeply and have fun!

LOVE POTION

Ok ok, there is really no such thing as a "love potion" in the fairytale, witch's brew sense. Regardless, this aromatic blend of neroli, jasmine, and rose oil creates a wonderfully feminine, floral combination that is perfect to relax and uplift any setting, and promote feelings of love.

Ingredients:

★ 3 drops of neroli oil
★ 2 drops of jasmine oil
★ 2 drops of rose oil
★ 100 ml of water

Instructions: Fill the diffuser container with fresh water (straight from the tap, or distilled or filtered, depending on preference). Add the drops of neroli, jasmine, and rose, then plug in the diffuser and turn it on at the desired setting.

For additional consideration: Like we said, there's no magic powers involved here - though it may feel like there are! After a few short minutes of diffusing this lovely blend, you'll be feeling at your fun, flirty best - and more than a little lovable!

THE SCENT OF SEDUCTION

Best to keep this blend in a space frequented by adults only - it's about to get sultry in here! This special recipe is laced with some of nature's sexiest aromas, all working together to support your body's hormone balance and energy levels. For those who might be trying for a baby, the life-giving strawflower oil (better known in medicinal circles as "Immortelle" or the "Everlasting Daisy") and ovary-stimulating ginger in this recipe can only help your chances!

Ingredients:

★ 2 drops of jasmine oil

★ 2 drops of strawflower oil

★ 1 drop of rose oil

★ 2 drops of neroli oil

★ 2 drops of ginger oil

★ 100 ml of water

Instructions: Fill the diffuser container with fresh water (straight from the tap, or distilled or filtered, depending on preference). Add the drops of jasmine, neroli, strawflower, rose, and ginger oil, then plug in the diffuser and turn it on at the desired setting.

For additional consideration: On your own or enjoyed with company, this blend will release a relaxed, invigorating blend from your diffuser, and leave you at your most physically confident and attractive. Have fun with this blend, and feel free to tinker with the ratios. This blend is all about your body's desires, so go with it!

AROMATIC APHRODISIAC

Here's another blend that's best not to use around children. For when it's more than just a little romance you've got on your mind, this sensual blend of sandalwood, anise, jasmine, and ylang-ylang is the perfect way to set the mood for physical love.

Ingredients:

★ 5 drops of sandalwood oil
★ I drop of anise oil
★ I drop of jasmine oil
★ I drop of ylang-ylang oil
★ I00 ml of water

Instructions: Fill the diffuser container with fresh water (straight from the tap, or distilled or filtered, depending on preference). Add the drops of sandalwood, anise, jasmine, and ylang-ylang, then plug in the diffuser and turn it on at the desired setting.

For additional consideration: Let this blend enter your senses and arouse your spirit. In no time at all these sensual aromas will stimulate you and your partner from head to toe, perfect for enhanced intimacy and truly intense experience.

EASY, TIGER

Sometimes, the last thing you want is an aphrodisiac — and for some, an overactive libido can be a real problem, preventing people from focusing on work, family, hobbies, or other joys and responsibilities in life. This blend of cooling, calming marjoram, anise, ho wood, and spearmint is the perfect blend to relax one's body — and tame that libido, so as to carry on with the rest of life.

Ingredients:
★ 2 drops of marjoram oil
★ 1 drop of anise oil
★ 100 ml of water
★ 2 drops of ho wood
★ 1 drop of spearmint oil

Instructions: Fill the diffuser container with fresh water (straight from the tap, or distilled or filtered, depending on preference). Add the drops of marjoram, ho wood, anise and spearmint oil, then plug in the diffuser and turn it on at the desired setting.

For additional consideration: This blend is made up of oils that are known for promoting peace and calm in your body. Use this blend to help clear your mind and focus on necessary tasks before you play.

DEEP SLEEP SLEEPY TIME

Sleep is just about the most important physical process our bodies go through on a regular basis – with the possible exception of breathing. Nothing else quite heals and repairs your system, helps fight off disease and ailments, and promotes overall well being like a good night's sleep. This powerful blend of chamomile, clary sage, and bergamot at bedtime will promote a deep and restful slumber – and all the benefits it brings.

Ingredients:

★ 4 drops of chamomile oil

★ 2 drops of bergamot oil

★ 2 drops of clary sage oil

★ 100 ml of water

Instructions: Fill the diffuser container with fresh water (straight from the tap, or distilled or filtered, depending on preference). Add the drops of chamomile, clary sage, and bergamot, then plug in the diffuser and turn it on at the desired setting.

For additional consideration: Breathe deeply and let this blend lull you into a profoundly restful state, perfect to fall asleep and stay asleep through the night. Wake up feeling refreshed and rejuvenated!

SPIRIT

Attitude, Faith, Personal Disposition and Relationships, Love, and Emotional Well Being.

Our moods, instincts, emotions, and feelings for ourselves and others are all guided by the limbic system — an intricate network of nerves and systems in the brain that guides everything from pleasure and anger to nurturing and appetite. Also known as the "paleomammalian brain," the limbic system controls our most primal selves, and its' balanced and healthy functioning is inextricably linked to daily well being.

When our primal functions of fear, anger, or grief are activated, our hormonal and nervous networks must be able to process appropriately to move forward in balance. Without that balance, these basic drives can become thwarted and lead to anxiety, rage, or depression. The good news is that nature has given us the power to restore balance — most effectively, through our sense of smell, that prehistoric guide for life and survival.

Similarly, our basic instincts for love, affection, pleasure seeking or joy can be nurtured, enhanced, and rewarded with the right stimuli, *and there is no better way to do so than through aromatherapy. Scents and fragrances unlock the connections deep within the limbic system to help our emotions and feelings remain in balance.*

The cool mist diffusion recipes in this section are all designed to stimulate various areas of that complex limbic network for optimal balance and function in a range of circumstances. From the mood stabilizing properties of geranium oil to the soulful serenity that comes from angelica extract, these blends demystify the ancient and spiritual aspects of our feeling, loving, laughing, praying and playing selves.

FRESH AND FREE

Nothing frees the spirits quite like a few deep breaths of fresh air - and nothing freshens stale air like this powerful blend of citrus aromas. As lovely as is this blend is for the senses, it does even more to lift the mood - so pop these scents in your diffuser and set your spirit free!

Ingredients:

★ 3 drops of orange oil

★ 2 drops of grapefruit oil

★ 2 drops of lime oil

★ 1 drop of lemon oil

★ 100 ml of water

Instructions: Fill the diffuser container with fresh water (straight from the tap, or distilled or filtered, depending on preference). Add the drops of orange, grapefruit, lime, and lemon, then plug in the diffuser and turn it on at the desired setting.

For additional consideration: Before you know it, this diffusion blend will have your air feeling cleaner and fresher - and your spirits lighter with every breath. Inhale deeply and enjoy the uplifting effects of this powerful citrus combination.

SPRING TIME

Maybe you need a little extra boost to enjoy springtime - or maybe it's the dead of winter and you want to create that light, airy feel that comes with spring. Either way, this bright and floral blend of cedarwood, ylang-ylang and jasmine will have you feeling sunnier in no time.

Ingredients:

★ 4 drops of cedarwood oil

★ 2 drops of ylang-ylang oil

★ 2 drops of jasmine oil

★ 100 ml of water

Instructions: Fill the diffuser container with fresh water (straight from the tap, or distilled or filtered, depending on preference). Add the drops of cedarwood, ylang-ylang, and jasmine, then plug in the diffuser and turn it on at the desired setting.

For additional consideration: Whatever the weather, this blend will quite literally put spring in the air in mere moments. With a few deep breaths, you'll feel sunnier and your mood lighter - perfect to enjoy a spring day, or simply the feeling of one.

BLOSSOM BLEND

Life got you down? Feeling a little worse for wear? This beautifully floral aroma with citrus undertones is perfect to lift the spirits and rejuvenate the senses. Like a flower blossoming in the spring, your mood will brighten and lift, leaving you feeling beautiful and fresh inside and out.

Ingredients:

★ 3 drops of jasmine oil
★ 3 drops of patchouli oil
★ 2 drops of lemon oil
★ 100 ml of water

Instructions: Fill the diffuser container with fresh water (straight from the tap, or distilled or filtered, depending on preference). Add the drops of jasmine, patchouli, and lemon, then plug in the diffuser and turn it on at the desired setting.

For additional consideration: No matter the season, this blend will bring the essence of spring into your space, soothing and lifting your spirits and brightening even the darkest day. Breathe deeply and smile, knowing that you're doing yourself a wonderful, aromatic favor.

UNWIND

We all need to give ourselves permission to let go and relax
sometimes mentally, physically, and even emotionally. This blend of
calming lavender, chamomile, and clary sage, with uplifting ylang-
ylang and relaxing geranium, is the perfect aromatic combination to
help that healing and unwinding process begin.

Ingredients:

★ 2 drops of lavender oil
★ 1 drop of chamomile oil
★ 1 drop of ylang-ylang oil

★ 2 drops of geranium oil
★ 1 drop of clary sage oil
★ 100 ml of water

Instructions: Fill the diffuser container with fresh water (straight
from the tap, or distilled or filtered, depending on preference). Add the
drops of lavender, geranium, chamomile, clary sage, and ylang-ylang,
then plug in the diffuser and turn it on at the desired setting.

For additional consideration: This is an excellent blend to diffuse after
a long week. There truly is nothing more wonderful than giving yourself a chance to unwind and relax. This blend in your diffuser will
help you do just that.

HAPPY HOUR

No cocktails needed to get this party started! This aromatic mix of lime and peppermint is the perfect way to add pep to any space. Whether you're actually hosting a party, or if you just want to feel like you are, this is a great blend to lighten the mood and lift the spirits.

Ingredients:

★ 5 drops of lime oil
★ 3 drops of peppermint oil
★ 100 ml of water

Instructions: Fill the diffuser container with fresh water (straight from the tap, or distilled or filtered, depending on preference). Add the drops of lime and peppermint, then plug in the diffuser and turn it on at the desired setting.

For additional consideration: This zingy blend will put a spring in your step and brighten your mood, perfect to create a festive party atmosphere from the inside out. A few deep inhales and you'll be ready to party down in no time!

SUMMER RAIN

You know those hot, sweaty summer days when you pray for rain, and
finally it comes - cool, refreshing, and calming with all the power of
Mother Nature? This deceptively simple blend of lemon and vetiver
essential oils does just that...with or without actual rain.

Ingredients:

★ 4 drops of lemon oil
★ 2 drops of vetiver oil
★ 100 ml of water

Instructions: Fill the diffuser container with fresh water (straight from
the tap, or distilled or filtered, depending on preference). Add the drops
of lemon and vetiver, then plug in the diffuser and turn it on at the desired setting.

For additional consideration: This is an energizing and refreshing blend
that will balance and calm not only the spirit, but the body and mind
as well. Take several long, deep breaths and feel your mood cool and
refresh, just as if you're being showered in that welcome rain on a hot
summer's day!

ANGELIC CALM

This simple recipe contains extract of the delicate flowering herb angelica, sometimes referred to as the "oil of angels" for its ability to soothe jangled nerves and stimulate happy memories. It's paired here with geranium essence, which is also known for its stress relieving properties along with its overall balancing effect.

Ingredients:

★ 3 drops of angelica oil
★ 2 drops of geranium oil
★ 100 ml of water

Instructions: Fill the diffuser container with fresh water (straight from the tap, or distilled or filtered, depending on preference). Add the drops of angelica and geranium, then plug in the diffuser and turn it on at the desired setting.

For additional consideration: This blend works wonders day or night, so feel free to use any time you need a touch of heavenly calm or a gentle mood lift. This diffusion is a great way to give yourself a little dose of comfort that will go a long way.

NATURAL UPLIFT

This powerful, fruity blend is the perfect aromatic combination to help invigorate a low mood. And, if you're already having a pleasant day, this blend will help make it even better, with invigorating grapefruit, jasmine, and delightful ylang-ylang. Use this blend any time you want to add a natural lift to your day!

Ingredients:

* ★ 3 drops of grapefruit oil
* ★ I drop of ylang-ylang oil
* ★ I drop of jasmine oil
* ★ IOO ml of water

Instructions: Fill the diffuser container with fresh water (straight from the tap, or distilled or filtered, depending on preference). Add the drops of grapefruit, jasmine, and ylang-ylang, then plug in the diffuser and turn it on at the desired setting.

For additional consideration: A few deep breaths of this fruity blend, and you'll feel your spirits start to lift. As you exhale, visualize expelling any negative thoughts and energy, and as you inhale take in all the goodness that nature has to offer.

CHASING THE BLUES AWAY

No matter what the circumstances, all of us suffer from the blues from time to time - when it feels like an endless downpour, even when the skies are bright. For those unhappy times, give this diffusion blend a try, and see if this uplifting, soothing blend of bergamot, lavender and clary sage doesn't chase those blues away.

Ingredients:

★ 3 drops of bergamot oil

★ 2 drops of clary sage oil

★ 2 drops of lavender oil

★ 100 ml of water

Instructions: Fill the diffuser container with fresh water (straight from the tap, or distilled or filtered, depending on preference). Add the drops of bergamot, lavender, and clary sage, then plug in the diffuser and turn it on at the desired setting.

For additional consideration: This is the perfect diffusion to brighten your day any time you're feeling a little blue, so just close your eyes, breathe deeply, and let these energizing, gently uplifting natural aromas work their magic.

FULL MOON

A full moon will amplify whatever is going on in your body, your mind, and your spirit. Use this clarifying and inspiring blend to harness the positive energy of the full moon, and to let go of any negative energies you may be hanging onto.

Ingredients:

★ 3 drops of cedarwood oil

★ 2 drops of juniper berry oil

★ 2 drops of cypress oil

★ 1 drop of lime oil

★ 100 ml of water

Instructions: Fill the diffuser container with fresh water (straight from the tap, or distilled or filtered, depending on preference). Add the drops of cedarwood, juniper berry, cypress, and lime, then plug in the diffuser and turn it on at the desired setting.

For additional consideration: The cypress and cedarwood in this blend are grounding and stabilizing, while the hint of lime and the emotionally stimulating juniper berry are the perfect complements to heighten your sensations to harness all the positive power of the full moon.

ENTERTAIN

Whether you're planning a raucous party or a sedate gathering, this uplifting yet soothing blend of bergamot, geranium, and lavender will create the perfect atmosphere to help loosen up your guests and ensure everyone has a great time.

Ingredients:

★ 4 drops of bergamot oil
★ 2 drops of geranium oil
★ 2 drops of lavender oil
★ 100 ml of water

Instructions: Fill the diffuser container with fresh water (straight from the tap, or distilled or filtered, depending on preference). Add the drops of bergamot, geranium, and lavender, then plug in the diffuser and turn it on at the desired setting.

For additional consideration: In a matter of minutes, this blend will fill your space with the perfect aromatic setting to get everyone in the mood for socializing. Breathe deeply and smile knowing that your event is sure to be a sweet smelling success!

STRESS BE GONE

This recipe combines the balancing, stress relieving duo of lavender and cypress, both excellent oils for stabilizing both body and mood. Cypress can be especially helpful for those dealing with long term stressors or past traumas, and the rosemary in this blend supports overall support and strength for body, mind and spirit alike.

Ingredients:

* 3 drops of lavender oil
* 2 drops of rosemary oil
* 3 drops of cypress oil
* 100 ml of water

Instructions: Fill the diffuser container with fresh water (straight from the tap, or distilled or filtered, depending on preference). Add the drops of lavender, cypress, and rosemary, then plug in the diffuser and turn it on at the desired setting.

For additional consideration: This recipe provides a good balance of both relaxation and energy, meaning it's appropriate to use any time of day. This is the blend to use when you need some extra help to relax and take care of yourself.

ANXIETY AWAY

Chamomile is loved around the world for its quieting effect on the nerves. It blends perfectly with angelica oil for a powerful anxiety reducing recipe, bolstered by cheering mandarin and just a hint of grounding basil. This is the perfect mix for those days when you need a little support to keep your worries from getting the best of you.

Ingredients:

★ 3 drops of roman chamomile oil   ★ 3 drops of angelica oil

★ 2 drops of mandarin oil   ★ 1 drop of basil oil

★ 100 ml of water

Instructions: Fill the diffuser container with fresh water (straight from the tap, or distilled or filtered, depending on preference). Add the drops of roman chamomile, angelica, mandarin, and basil, then plug in the diffuser and turn it on at the desired setting.

For additional consideration: This blend is best to use in the late afternoon or evenings, as it is likely to produce a deeply relaxed state. These aromas are ideal for the end of a long day at work, when you nerves could use some soothing special care.

STRESS RELIEVER

This light and floral blend, with a hint of woody undertones, is the perfect way to breathe away your troubles. The lavender, geranium and ylang-ylang are particularly effective in soothing the nerves, and the sandalwood and bergamot will restore a sense of balance and stability to your spirits.

Ingredients:

- ★ 3 drops of lavender oil
- ★ 2 drops of ylang-ylang oil
- ★ 1 drop of bergamot oil
- ★ 2 drops of geranium oil
- ★ 1 drop of sandalwood oil
- ★ 100 ml of water

Instructions: Fill the diffuser container with fresh water (straight from the tap, or distilled or filtered, depending on preference). Add the drops of lavender, geranium, ylang-ylang, sandalwood, and bergamot, then plug in the diffuser and turn it on at the desired setting.

For additional consideration: With a few deep inhales, this diffusion will start to relieve any emotional stress and help to center the chaos of a busy and overworked mind. Breathe in and enjoy the sense of calm that these aromas will bring.

SPIRIT REVITALIZER

Are you longing for Friday.. on Tuesday? Are you counting the minutes until your next break, or nap? Are you daydreaming when you're supposed to be doing something productive? Don't wish your week away — instead give your spirit a lift with this simple yet powerful blend of revitalizing basil and spearmint.

Ingredients:

★ 3 drops of basil oil
★ 3 drops of spearmint oil
★ 100 ml of water

Instructions: Fill the diffuser container with fresh water (straight from the tap, or distilled or filtered, depending on preference). Add the drops of basil and spearmint, then plug in the diffuser and turn it on at the desired setting.

For additional consideration: This is a wonderful blend to use first thing in the morning, or throughout the day until early afternoon. It will help stimulate alertness and clarity, so it's best not to use it in the evenings too close to bedtime. Breathe deeply, and revel in the refreshing lift of this wonderful aromatic blend!

MAN CAVE

Maybe the man of the house needs a space that truly feels like it's his own — or maybe you just want to give your home a masculine scent and feel. Whatever the impetus, the combination of cedarwood, cypress, and wintergreen in this blend is the perfect blend to create a strong, grounding, masculine atmosphere.

Ingredients:
★ 3 drops of cedarwood oil
★ 3 drops of cypress oil
★ 3 drops of wintergreen oil
★ 100 ml of water

Instructions: Fill the diffuser container with fresh water (straight from the tap, or distilled or filtered, depending on preference). Add the drops of cedarwood, cypress, and wintergreen, then plug in the diffuser and turn it on at the desired setting.

For additional consideration: This masculine and woody blend of aromas will have your diffuser taking pride of place in the man cave or it will simply create one out of any space! Breathe deeply and enjoy the strength and grounding balance this diffusion provides.

SUMMER BREEZE

You know the gentle, cooling calm that comes over you when a warm summer breeze ruffles your hair and caresses your skin? That's pretty much exactly what this blend of peppermint, orange, and lemongrass feels like – from the inside out, and with no actual summertime required!

Ingredients:

★ 4 drops of orange oil

★ 2 drops of lemongrass oil

★ 2 drops of peppermint oil

★ 100 ml of water

Instructions: Fill the diffuser container with fresh water (straight from the tap, or distilled or filtered, depending on preference). Add the drops of orange, peppermint, and lemongrass, then plug in the diffuser and turn it on at the desired setting.

For additional consideration: This refreshing blend is the perfect combination of aromas to cool the mind and body, while lifting the spirits with the sunny scents of long summer days and gentle breezes. Breathe deeply and feel yourself growing lighter and more relaxed with every inhale.

ROSE GARDEN

Maybe no one ever promised you that life would be a rose garden but you can create the atmosphere of one right in your own home, or any other space, with this wonderful, heady floral blend reminiscent of a rose garden in full bloom.

Ingredients:

★ 3 drops of lime oil

★ 3 drops of bergamot oil

★ 1 drop of ylang-ylang oil

★ 1 drop of rose oil

★ 100 ml of water

Instructions: Fill the diffuser container with fresh water (straight from the tap, or distilled or filtered, depending on preference). Add the drops of lime, bergamot, ylang-ylang, and rose, then plug in the diffuser and turn it on at the desired setting.

For additional consideration: This wonderful blend is sure to lift your spirits with just a few breaths, with this aromatic combination of floral scents that will help you focus on the beauty around you. Inhale deeply and enjoy the sensation of your very own rose garden and don't be surprised if life doesn't feel just a little more wonderful.

HAPPY MIST

This recipe is wonderful for all around mood support. The citrus bouquet contains oils known for their refreshing and detoxifying properties, as well as their emotionally uplifting effects. The bergamot blends in perfectly, adding a steady energy boost and a sense of allday rejuvenating calm.

Ingredients:

★ 2 drops of wild orange oil
★ 2 drops of lemon oil
★ 2 drops of bergamot oil
★ 100 ml of water

Instructions: Fill the diffuser container with fresh water (straight from the tap, or distilled or filtered, depending on preference). Add the drops of wild orange, lemon, and bergamot, then plug in the diffuser and turn it on at the desired setting.

For additional consideration: Breathe deeply and enjoy the feeling of happy contentment that comes with this cheerful mix. This is a great blend to use in your diffuser any time of day, though best to avoid before bed time due to its invigorating effects.

BREATHE JOY

This energizing and cheering blend will lift the mood in any space. The bergamot and ylang-ylang work together to promote a positive attitude and can do energy. Bergamot is an especially strong support to sensations of joy, making the simple things in life that much more pleasurable. The grapefruit adds a rejuvenating zest to the blend that makes this recipe a hit in the home or office.

Ingredients:

★ 4 drops of bergamot oil   ★ 2 drops of ylang-ylang oil

★ I drop of grapefruit oil   ★ IOO ml of water

Instructions: Fill the diffuser container with fresh water (straight from the tap, or distilled or filtered, depending on preference). Add the drops of bergamot, ylang-ylang, and grapefruit, then plug in the diffuser and turn it on at the desired setting.

For additional consideration: This blend is best for mornings or day time, as it lends a sustained rejuvenating uplift to a space. Breathe deeply and enjoy...and find yourself spreading that joy to others around you throughout the day!

CHIRPING CHEERFUL

This blend in the diffuser is like having a bright spring day in the air with all the hope and optimism that brings. Even during the cold winter months, the balanced mix of geranium, frankincense, and wild orange will promote a sense of sunny positivity and grounded optimism.

Ingredients:

★ 3 drops of wild orange oil

★ 3 drops of frankincense oil

★ 2 drops of geranium oil

★ 100 ml of water

Instructions: Fill the diffuser container with fresh water (straight from the tap, or distilled or filtered, depending on preference). Add the drops of wild orange, frankincense, and geranium, then plug in the diffuser and turn it on at the desired setting.

For additional consideration: The lighter geranium ratio in this blend keeps the aroma from being too floral, which makes this recipe an excellent choice for office diffusion. And who couldn't use a little extra cheering up at the workplace? With this recipe, everyone can benefit.

GRACE AND GRATITUDE

Grace and gratitude aren't just feelings or states - they are practices, like yoga for the soul that open us up to a kinder, gentler world, allowing us to give as much goodness as we take in and vice versa. This warm and up-lifting blend of bergamot, grapefruit, ylang-ylang, frankincense, cypress, and ginger creates the perfect sensory atmosphere to focus on these joy giving practices and fill your senses, spirit and mind with grace and gratitude.

Ingredients:

★ 2 drops of bergamot oil

★ 2 drops of grapefruit oil

★ 1 drop of ylang-ylang oil

★ 1 drop of frankincense oil

★ 1 drop of cypress oil

★ 1 drop of ginger oil

★ 100 ml of water

Instructions: Fill the diffuser container with fresh water (straight from the tap, or distilled or filtered, depending on preference). Add the drops of bergamot, grapefruit, ylang-ylang, frankincense, cypress, and ginger, then plug in the diffuser and turn it on at the desired setting.

For additional consideration: Take a moment with this diffusion to close your eyes, breathe in deeply, and visualize all the people and things in life for which you're grateful. When you open your eyes, you might just find that the world is that much more beautiful a place. Enjoy and carry on with a wonderful day.

PERSONAL PICK-ME-UP

The sandalwood, rose, and bergamot in this recipe are a powerful mood elevating trio. Lavender soothes any hurt feelings while the rose and sandalwood stabilize the hormones and balance the emotions. This is a wonderful recipe for turning around a gloomy day.

Ingredients:

★ 3 drops of bergamot oil
★ 2 drops of rose oil
★ 3 drops of sandalwood oil
★ 100 ml of water

Instructions: Fill the diffuser container with fresh water (straight from the tap, or distilled or filtered, depending on preference). Add the drops of bergamot, rose, and sandalwood, then plug in the diffuser and turn it on at the desired setting.

For additional consideration: This blend is mellow enough to use in the evenings, though it also works great for daytime use. These aromas are a comforting addition to any space, so breathe deeply and feel better.

TRANQUILITY

The lime and ho wood in this relaxing blend both as powerful calmants. The lime adds a refreshing and uplifting twist, creating the perfect combination of fragrances to diffuse for those days when you could use a little extra serenity in your mood.

Ingredients:
★ 3 drops of lime oil
★ 2 drops of vetiver oil
★ 2 drops of ho wood oil
★ 100 ml of water

Instructions: Fill the diffuser container with fresh water (straight from the tap, or distilled or filtered, depending on preference). Add the drops of lime, vetiver, and ho wood, then plug in the diffuser and turn it on at the desired setting.

For additional consideration: This calming blend will help balance the mind and promote a deep sense of inner tranquility with every breath. Relax and smile, knowing that you are emotionally stable regardless of the chaos that may be surrounding you.

COMFORT

The combination of soothing lavender and ho wood, uplifting ylang-ylang and cedarwood, and the overall well being benefits of orange in this wonderful mix are as comforting as a warm blanket. Diffuse this blend anytime you could use a little aromatic tender loving care.

Ingredients:

★ 3 drops of orange oil

★ 2 drops of ho wood oil

★ 1 drop of cedarwood oil

★ 2 drops of lavender oil

★ 1 drop of ylang-ylang oil

★ 100 ml of water

Instructions: Fill the diffuser container with fresh water (straight from the tap, or distilled or filtered, depending on preference). Add the drops of orange, lavender, ho wood, ylang-ylang, and cedarwood, then plug in the diffuser and turn it on at the desired setting.

For additional consideration: A few deep inhales of this blend will leave you feeling as comforted as if you were in front of a hot fire on a cold winter's night, or receiving a hug from a loved one at the end of a long hard day. Breathe in and let these aromas comfort you mind, body, and most of all...your spirit.

BREAK-UP BLEND

Not all relationships are destined for the altar. Break ups happen to the best of us, for any number of reasons. This grounding, enlightening blend of bergamot, rosemary, peppermint, and white fir is an excellent diffusion to help clear yourself of any negative energy and move forward positively.

Ingredients:

★ 2 drops of bergamot oil

★ 2 drops of rosemary oil

★ 2 drops of peppermint oil

★ 1 drop of white fir oil

★ 100 ml of water

Instructions: Fill the diffuser container with fresh water (straight from the tap, or distilled or filtered, depending on preference). Add the drops of bergamot, rosemary, peppermint, and white fir, then plug in the diffuser and turn it on at the desired setting.

For additional consideration: These aromas will create the perfect fragrance combination to help you put things into perspective, and encourage you to work through a respectful and empathetic break up.

CHAKRA BALANCE

The chakra energies in our bodies are still disputed by Western medicine, but in Eastern practice they are long known to have a powerful effect on our emotional, physical, and spiritual health. The grounding frankincense, uplifting clary sage and healing jasmine in this blend create the perfect aromatic combination to open and balance your chakras for the benefit of your whole system.

Ingredients:

★ 4 drops of frankincense oil
★ 2 drops of jasmine oil
★ 2 drops of clary sage oil
★ 100 ml of water

Instructions: Fill the diffuser container with fresh water (straight from the tap, or distilled or filtered, depending on preference). Add the drops of frankincense, clary sage, and jasmine, then plug in the diffuser and turn it on at the desired setting.

For additional consideration: This diffusion will have your chakra centers feeling balanced, open, and empowered within just a few minutes, thus improving your overall sense of vitality, emotional stability, and physical wellbeing. Breathe deeply, and enjoy!

SOOTHING SCENTS

This blend of calming chamomile and vetiver, uplifting frankincense and luxurious rose is the perfect fragrance combination to ease whatever emotions may be troubling you. Enjoy this wonderful diffusion and let the subtle aromas soothe your very soul.

Ingredients:

★ 2 drops of chamomile oil

★ 2 drops of vetiver oil

★ 2 drops of frankincense oil

★ I drop of rose oil

★ I00 ml of water

Instructions: Fill the diffuser container with fresh water (straight from the tap, or distilled or filtered, depending on preference). Add the drops of chamomile, vetiver, frankincense, and rose, then plug in the diffuser and turn it on at the desired setting.

For additional consideration: Even if you can only take a moment or two to stop and acknowledge this blend, you will find it even more beneficial. It is a beautifully mellow aroma that will gently calm your whole system from the inside out.

INNER STRENGTH

We all face challenges in life and, sometimes, our resilience may need a little boost to help get us through. For those difficult times, try this empowering blend of basil, bergamot, cinnamon, lemon and black pepper that will help summon your inner reserves and proceed with true emotional strength.

Ingredients:

★ 2 drops of basil oil

★ 1 drop of cinnamon oil

★ 1 drop of black pepper oil

★ 2 drops of bergamot oil

★ 1 drop of lemon oil

★ 100 ml of water

Instructions: Fill the diffuser container with fresh water (straight from the tap, or distilled or filtered, depending on preference). Add the drops of basil, bergamot, cinnamon, lemon, and black pepper, then plug in the diffuser and turn it on at the desired setting.

For additional consideration: This is a wonderful blend to diffuse when the obstacles in front of you seem insurmountable. After just a few deep breaths, you may find yourself surprised at what you can overcome.

MEDITATION MIST

Meditation is a wonderful way to nourish the soul, calm the mind, and even heal the body with the power of a peaceful, powerful emotional state. This blend of lavender, sandalwood, frankincense, and ylang-ylang is my go to diffusion for my own meditation practice. It is perfect for helping to clear my mind and focus on stillness, breath, and peace.

Ingredients:

★ 3 drops of sandalwood oil

★ 2 drops of lavender oil

★ 100 ml of water

★ 3 drops of frankincense oil

★ 1 drop of ylang-ylang oil

Instructions: Fill the diffuser container with fresh water (straight from the tap, or distilled or filtered, depending on preference). Add the drops of lavender, sandalwood, frankincense, and ylang-ylang, then plug in the diffuser and turn it on at the desired setting.

For additional consideration: This peaceful blend will help calm and center the mind with just a few breaths. It's not only perfect to use during meditation, but also any time you simply wish to clear your mind and steady your emotional state.

BREATHE IN BALANCE

Some days the emotions just feel out of whack, plain and simple. Up seems down, happy seems angry, and everything is topsy turvy inside for no apparent reason. For those days, I can't recommend anything more than this balancing blend of soothing lavender and patchouli, grounding bergamot, and uplifting ylang-ylang. Breathe in and let the sense of balance find you.

Ingredients:

★ 2 drops of lavender oil
★ 2 drops of patchouli oil
★ 100 ml of water
★ 2 drops of bergamot oil
★ 2 drops of ylang-ylang

Instructions: Fill the diffuser container with fresh water (straight from the tap, or distilled or filtered, depending on preference). Add the drops of lavender, bergamot, patchouli, and ylang-ylang, then plug in the diffuser and turn it on at the desired setting.

For additional consideration: This is the ideal blend to use when your thoughts and emotions are all over the place. With a few deep breaths of this balancing blend, you'll feel evened out in no time.

HAPPY THOUGHTS

The sweet orange blossom bestows its blessings in spades with the neroli oil in this good vibes inducing recipe. Accented with lemon and grapefruit oils, this blend refreshes both the mind and the mood and stimulates the mind towards proactive and life affirming thinking.

Ingredients:

★ 4 drops of neroli oil
★ 2 drops of lemon oil
★ 2 drops of grapefruit oil
★ 100 ml of water

Instructions: Fill the diffuser container with fresh water (straight from the tap, or distilled or filtered, depending on preference). Add the drops of neroli, lemon, and grapefruit, then plug in the diffuser and turn it on at the desired setting.

For additional consideration: This blend is fine to use anytime you want to encourage a more positive train of thought. It will perk up any case of morning "blahs," and when used in the evenings may stimulate the kind of happy thoughts that will lead to sweet dreams.

SCENTS OF SIMPLICITY

"Simplify your life." It's such easy advice to give, which perhaps is why it's so common, yet so difficult to follow! This clean, refreshing blend of lemon, rosemary, and cypress oils is the perfect diffusion to help you to not sweat the small stuff and focus on what matters, and leave the rest behind.

Ingredients:

★ 3 drops of lemon oil
★ 2 drops of rosemary oil
★ 1 drop of cypress oil
★ 100 ml of water

Instructions: Fill the diffuser container with fresh water (straight from the tap, or distilled or filtered, depending on preference). Add the drops of lemon, rosemary, and cypress, then plug in the diffuser and turn it on at the desired setting.

For additional consideration: This blend is particularly perfect for when you're facing an overwhelmingly complex day. Let these scents help you pare back to what's important, and find ways to simplify your life.

MOTIVATION BLEND

This is the perfect combination of fragrances for those times when you know what needs to be done, and you just need the will to do it. The sharp zing of black pepper, along with bracing lime, frankincense, and refreshing orange, will help get you started and keep you going whatever the task!

Ingredients:

★ 3 drops of black pepper oil

★ 3 drops of lime oil

★ 3 drops of orange oil

★ 1 drop of frankincense oil

★ 100 ml of water

Instructions: Fill the diffuser container with fresh water (straight from the tap, or distilled or filtered, depending on preference). Add the drops of black pepper, lime, orange, and frankincense, then plug in the diffuser and turn it on at the desired setting.

For additional consideration: Before you know it, this blend will have you raring to tackle that to do list, confront those demons, or just pursue whatever it is that you need to do that day. Breathe deeply and go forth!

GROUNDING GRACE

The combination of balance inducing vetiver with calming chamomile and sandalwood creates the perfect aromatic blend to keep your thoughts and feelings focused, centered, and grounded. This relaxing blend is ideal to help anchor your emotions and put you in the best possible spirit for whatever the day brings.

Ingredients:

- ★ 4 drops of vetiver oil
- ★ 2 drops of chamomile oil
- ★ 4 drops of sandalwood oil
- ★ 100 ml of water

Instructions: Fill the diffuser container with fresh water (straight from the tap, or distilled or filtered, depending on preference). Add the drops of vetiver, chamomile, and sandalwood, then plug in the diffuser and turn it on at the desired setting.

For additional consideration: This diffusion is an absolute godsend when I feel like I'm being pulled in too many different directions. A few deep inhales of these wonderful aromas, and my thoughts and feelings are centered once again, leaving me grounded and at my best.

POSITIVE PEP

Patchouli is a well known mood lifter, thanks to the essential oil's ability to lessen negative feelings, particularly disappointment. It also eases tension and promotes the sense of ease and comfort. In this recipe, the patchouli's power is enhanced by emotionally balancing bergamot and uplifting geranium.

Ingredients:

★ 3 drops of patchouli oil
★ 2 drops of bergamot oil
★ 2 drops of geranium oil
★ 100 ml of water

Instructions: Fill the diffuser container with fresh water (straight from the tap, or distilled or filtered, depending on preference). Add the drops of patchouli, bergamot, and geranium, then plug in the diffuser and turn it on at the desired setting.

For additional consideration: After just a few breaths of this cheering blend, you'll be feeling ready to embrace the day and whatever challenges it brings. Because the bergamot and geranium have a mild stimulating effect, this blend is best to enjoy during the day, not too close to bedtime

REASSURE AND RELAX

The ho wood and lavender in this blend are pure balm for the spirit and emotions. Combined with calming clary sage and uplifting, clarifying lemon in this mixture, you've got the perfect aromatic concoction to reassure and relax yourself, no matter what strife life may be throwing your way.

Ingredients:

★ 3 drops of clary sage oil   ★ 3 drops of lavender oil
★ 2 drops of ho wood oil   ★ 2 drops of lemon oil
★ 100 ml of water

Instructions: Fill the diffuser container with fresh water (straight from the tap, or distilled or filtered, depending on preference). Add the drops of clary sage, lavender, ho wood, and lemon, then plug in the diffuser and turn it on at the desired setting.

For additional consideration: This diffusion is an excellent choice when those daily stresses (or even major crises) threaten to overwhelm you. With a few deep breaths, this blend will have your mind and emotions feeling calmer and fresher in no time.

OPTIMISM BLEND

This recipe contains extract of calamus, a key ingredient in ayurvedic medicine due to its reparative properties and ability to calm and soothe both the nervous and limbic system. This recipe blends the healing calamus with healing clary sage and serenity stimulating tea tree oil, for an aroma that's both relaxing and inspiring, heralding good things to come.

Ingredients:

★ 3 drops of calamus oil
★ 2 drops of clary sage oil
★ 2 drops of tea tree oil
★ 100 ml of water

Instructions: Fill the diffuser container with fresh water (straight from the tap, or distilled or filtered, depending on preference). Add the drops of calamus, clary sage, and tea tree, then plug in the diffuser and turn it on at the desired setting.

For additional consideration: This recipe is not too stimulating for evening use, but it's especially beneficial in the morning or daytime, as it will help propel positive action and productive forward thinking.

SUNNY SIDE UP

Cinnamon has been used for millennia to help lighten moods, particularly during the long dark winter months. More recently, cinnamon was found in one study to reduce irritability among automobile drivers. This blend adds a touch of invigorating lemon and emotion balancing rosemary for the perfect aromatic day brightener.

Ingredients:

★ 5 drops of cinnamon oil

★ I drop of rosemary oil

★ 2 drops of lemon oil

★ IOO ml of water

Instructions: Fill the diffuser container with fresh water (straight from the tap, or distilled or filtered, depending on preference). Add the drops of cinnamon, lemon, and rosemary, then plug in the diffuser and turn it on at the desired setting.

For additional consideration: This invigorating blend is best to avoid before bedtime, as it will stimulate your creative and social energies. It's an excellent recipe to use in the workplace, to help spread those sunny feelings to your coworkers.

HARMONY BLEND

This combination of joyful patchouli, spicy cinnamon, and uplifting white fir and wintergreen creates an outstanding aromatic palate to optimize group or team work. Whether at home or at work, diffuse this blend any time you need to get people working together for the best possible outcome...in harmony!

Ingredients:

★ 3 drops of patchouli oil

★ 2 drops of cinnamon oil

★ 100 ml of water

★ 2 drops of white fir oil

★ I drop of wintergreen oil

Instructions: Fill the diffuser container with fresh water (straight from the tap, or distilled or filtered, depending on preference). Add the drops of patchouli, white fir, cinnamon, wintergreen, then plug in the diffuser and turn it on at the desired setting.

For additional consideration: Working together to achieve any goal is just a little easier (and better) with these grounding, revitalizing aromas. Diffuse and find that after a few minutes, you've created the perfect atmosphere for helping people to balance their energies and create harmony in the group.

AROMATHERAPEUTIC ANTI-DEPRESSIVE

Vanilla is a marvelous and all natural anti depressant, highly effective in lifting the mood and stimulating the body's own pleasure receptors. It also helps to drive away anxiety and feelings of sadness. A touch cleansing lemon and mood balancing sandalwood only enhance the effects of the vanilla for a sweet smelling route to good feelings.

Ingredients:

★ 5 drops of vanilla oil

★ 2 drops of lemon oil

★ 2 drops of sandalwood oil

★ 100 ml of water

Instructions: Fill the diffuser container with fresh water (straight from the tap, or distilled or filtered, depending on preference). Add the drops of vanilla, lemon, sandalwood, then plug in the diffuser and turn it on at the desired setting.

For additional consideration: This blend can be used day or night to help stave off the blues; as part of a daily regimen it's an effective way to keep depression at bay. Remember to take a few moments with every diffusion to close your eyes and enjoy the fragrances with several deep breaths. By the time you open your eyes, you may well have a smile on your face.

POSITIVITY PLUS

Sandalwood is not only an excellent stabilizing agent, its extract is also effective in minimizing negative feelings. The black pepper oil in this recipe adds an extra dose of rejuvenating energy, along with the grounding and calming essence of clary sage. This blend is a fragrant way to inject a steady jolt of optimism into a space.

Ingredients:

★ 4 drops of sandalwood oil

★ 1 drop of clary sage oil

★ 2 drops of black pepper oil

★ 100 ml of water

Instructions: Fill the diffuser container with fresh water (straight from the tap, or distilled or filtered, depending on preference). Add the drops of sandalwood, black pepper, and clary sage, then plug in the diffuser and turn it on at the desired setting.

For additional consideration: It won't take long for this blend to work its magic. Feel the uplifting aromas raise your spirits with every inhale. This recipe's invigorating properties are mild enough that it's fine to use in the afternoons, though probably not right before bedtime.

SPIRIT CLEANSE

The soul needs to be detoxified just like the body and the mind. That's where frankincense and wild orange truly shine, together purifying and refreshing the limbic system to clear out negative emotions and leave behind a sense of positivity and newness. With just a touch of geranium oil, this energizing blend is a fragrant and effective mood tonic.

Ingredients:

★ 3 drops of frankincense oil
★ I drop of geranium oil
★ 3 drops of wild orange oil
★ IOO ml of water

Instructions: Fill the diffuser container with fresh water (straight from the tap, or distilled or filtered, depending on preference). Add the drops of frankincense, wild orange, and geranium, then plug in the diffuser and turn it on at the desired setting.

For additional consideration : Frankincense is bracing in a wonderful way so it's best to reserve this diffusion for morning or daytime use. The wild orange adds a delightfully sweet twist to any space, so be sure to enjoy this blend, and the renewal of spirit that it brings.

BREATHE IN THE NOW

It's easy to say, not quite as simple to do: be present, live in the moment. With this rich and grounding blend of neroli, bergamot, and geranium in your diffuser, that crucial counsel just got a little easier. The neroli's sweet orange blossom extract is uplifting and will stimulate a sense of positivity and clarity, while the bergamot and geranium are wonderfully stabilizing, promoting balanced emotion and calm thought.

Ingredients:

★ 3 drops of neroli oil

★ 2 drops of bergamot oil

★ I drop of geranium oil

★ IOO ml of water

Instructions: Fill the diffuser container with fresh water (straight from the tap, or distilled or filtered, depending on preference). Add the drops of neroli, bergamot, and geranium, then plug in the diffuser and turn it on at the desired setting.

For additional consideration: This blend is best to use in the home, or in a space where you can expect a little privacy and space to enjoy these centering fragrances. Take several deep breaths, keeping your eyes open, and spend a few minutes simply appreciating your surroundings. Notice a heightened presence throughout the day.

SOOTHING SWEET

It's little surprise we love roses so much. Along with the beauty of their flowers and the healing properties of their essential oils, rose extract is also known to alleviate depression and reduce anxiety. With the stabilizing energy of ylang-ylang oil, this is a simple but powerful recipe to comfort and uplift.

Ingredients:

★ 5 drops of rose oil

★ 2 drops of ylang-ylang oil

★ 100 ml of water

Instructions: Fill the diffuser container with fresh water (straight from the tap, or distilled or filtered, depending on preference). Add the drops of rose and ylang-ylang, then plug in the diffuser and turn it on at the desired setting.

For additional consideration: Let this enriching blend fill your senses and warm your heart. Best to avoid just before bedtime, as the ylang-ylang is stimulating, though fine for afternoon diffusions. With just a few deep breaths, this recipe will increase overall well being and contentment.

TEAMWORK TONIC

This is a fantastic blend in any circumstance, but particularly in group situations. This collection of oils gathers scents that have been used since ancient times in tribal rituals, stimulating a deeply ingrained sense of cooperation and collaboration. The rosemary and frankincense in this blend are particularly helpful in supporting positive social feelings, while the neroli and sandalwood are both balancing and cheering.

Ingredients:

★ 2 drops of rosemary oil

★ 1 drop of rose oil

★ 1 drop of roman chamomile oil

★ 1 drop of frankincense oil

★ 100 ml of water

★ 1 drop of cedarwood oil

★ 1 drop of geranium oil

★ 1 drop of sandalwood oil

★ 1 drop of jasmine oil

Instructions: Fill the diffuser container with fresh water (straight from the tap, or distilled or filtered, depending on preference). Add the drops of rosemary, cedarwood, rose, geranium, roman chamomile, sandalwood, frankincense, and jasmine, then plug in the diffuser and turn it on at the desired setting.

For additional consideration: This blend will stimulate and energize a space, though the chamomile and lavender keep it mellow and gentle enough for afternoon diffusion. The recipe is appropriate to use both at home and in the office, as the floral accents are not be overpowering.

BREATH OF KINDNESS

This is another great recipe to use in group settings, and particularly with children. The wild orange and geranium oils soothe anxieties and promote feelings of empathy and goodwill. The palmarosa extract has the added benefit of being a calmant and stress-reliever, making this an ideal blend to use in any space where a strong sense of peace and harmony is desired.

Ingredients:

★ 4 drops of palmarosa oil

★ 1 drop of geranium oil

★ 2 drops of wild orange oil

★ 100 ml of water

Instructions: Fill the diffuser container with fresh water (straight from the tap, or distilled or filtered, depending on preference). Add the drops of palmarosa, wild orange, and geranium, then plug in the diffuser and turn it on at the desired setting.

For additional consideration: This blend is mellowing enough to use in the evenings, even with easily stimulated children. Day or night, this is a wonderful recipe to breathe in and enhance feelings of friendship and comradery.

CONFIDENT CONTENTMENT

Extract of lemongrass can be an effective mood stabilizer, and it's especially helpful in generating feelings of confidence and self esteem. In this recipe, lemongrass is perfectly balanced with juniper oil, which is known to even out emotional swings, along with soothing and luscious lavender.

Ingredients:

* 5 drops of lemongrass oil
* 2 drops of juniper oil
* 3 drops of lavender oil
* 100 ml of water

Instructions: Fill the diffuser container with fresh water (straight from the tap, or distilled or filtered, depending on preference). Add the drops of lemongrass, lavender, and juniper, then plug in the diffuser and turn it on at the desired setting.

For additional consideration: This blend is energizing enough for daytime use, but thanks to the lavender keeps a calm enough atmosphere for evening as well. Whenever you use it, enjoy the deep sense of contentment it nurtures, and the feelings of positivity for the self and others.

LOVE YOURSELF

This recipe is simple but powerful, and all but guaranteed to put a smile on your face and a skip in your step. The jasmine is an effective mood lifter, and has been shown to increase feelings of self worth and contentment. The grapefruit is both cleansing and rejuvenating, bringing all the cheering benefits of sunny citrus. This is a wonderful blend to use in any space where you want to treat yourself. It's like giving yourself an aromatic hug!

Ingredients:

★ 6 drops of jasmine oil
★ 3 drops of grapefruit oil
★ 100 ml of water

Instructions: Fill the diffuser container with fresh water (straight from the tap, or distilled or filtered, depending on preference). Add the drops of jasmine and grapefruit, then plug in the diffuser and turn it on at the desired setting.

For additional consideration: This recipe can be used day or night, in any setting, so breathe deeply and feel free to enjoy regularly. There's no faster route to happiness than treating yourself right, and this diffusion is a great place to start.

HAPPY HAPPY, JOY JOY

This recipe combines the joyous zest of wild orange oil with the irresistible aroma of extract of wintergreen. These fragrances together will enhance sensations of pleasure and optimism, and stimulate a full body sense of well being and joyful anticipation.

Ingredients:

★ 3 drops of wild orange oil

★ 3 drops of wintergreen oil

★ 100 ml of water

Instructions: Fill the diffuser container with fresh water (straight from the tap, or distilled or filtered, depending on preference). Add the drops of wild orange and wintergreen, then plug in the diffuser and turn it on at the desired setting.

For additional consideration: This is an invigorating blend, but mild enough to use in the evenings as well as the daytime. Take several long inhales and let the aromas fill your senses for a surefire way to inject a dose of happy joy into any space.

PERSONAL POWER

The cheering scent of mandarin oil is also an effective support for a more stable mood and calm nerves. It's enhanced in this recipe with balancing lemongrass extract, uplifting cinnamon and grounding cedarwood. This blend is ideal for those days when we need to summon our inner power and present our personal best to the world.

Ingredients:

★ 3 drops of mandarin oil
★ 3 drops of lemongrass oil
★ 2 drops of cinnamon oil
★ 2 drops of cedarwood oil
★ 100 ml of water

Instructions: Fill the diffuser container with fresh water (straight from the tap, or distilled or filtered, depending on preference). Add the drops of mandarin, lemongrass, cinnamon, and cedarwood, then plug in the diffuser and turn it on at the desired setting.

For additional consideration: This blend is fine for evening use, though most beneficial during the day when that harnessed inner power will have a chance to shine. With just a few deep breaths, you'll be feeling calm, confident, and ready to show your true value to the world.

GOOD GRIEF

Dealing with loss is one of the most common hardships in life, and it take its toll on the spirit. This recipe provides a soothing and restorative aromatic therapy to help you through those tough times, with anxiety reducing nutmeg and deeply comforting vanilla. The touch of peppermint in this blend adds and extra source of balance and balm, likely to stimulate warm memories and decrease feelings of loneliness.

Ingredients:
★ 3 drops of nutmeg oil
★ 2 drops of peppermint oil
★ 3 drops of vanilla oil
★ 100 ml of water

Instructions: Fill the diffuser container with fresh water (straight from the tap, or distilled or filtered, depending on preference). Add the drops of nutmeg, vanilla, and peppermint, then plug in the diffuser and turn it on at the desired setting.

For additional consideration: Grief can be a long road, and there is no timeline for moving on from a loss and feeling better. Let this recipe act as a companion in that journey. Take a few deep breaths and take solace in these healing aromas. Have faith that in time, this too shall pass.

HEALING SORROW

Similar to grief, feelings of sorrow are important to feel as a means of passing through and beyond difficult periods in our lives. Instead of trying to suppress feelings of sorrow or loss, try diffusing this soothing and cathartic blend that may help you work through those feelings in a positive way.

Ingredients:
* 3 drops of rose oil
* 1 drop of chamomile oil
* 1 drop of frankincense oil
* 100 ml of water
* 1 drop of bergamot oil
* 1 drop of clary sage oil
* 1 drop of sandalwood oil

Instructions: Fill the diffuser container with fresh water (straight from the tap, or distilled or filtered, depending on preference). Add the drops of rose, bergamot, chamomile, clary sage, frankincense, and sandalwood, then plug in the diffuser and turn it on at the desired setting.

For additional consideration: Sorrow is a natural part of life and makes the happy moments that much more joyful. Use this blend to reflect upon whatever sadness you're experiencing, and on every inhale visualize yourself taking in strength, and on every exhale visualize yourself releasing tension and negativity. Even if you don't feel happier, you will soon start to feel far more able to deal with your sad emotions in a positive way.

ANGER MANAGEMENT

We all know what it's like to get hot under the collar and to struggle with channeling feelings of anger or even rage. The extract of blue tansy in this recipe is extremely effective in helping to control impulsive feelings, along with being a powerful overall calmer and nerve relaxant. Blended here with soothing patchouli and uplifting tangerine and wild orange oils, this recipe is an excellent way to give yourself a chance to cool down and reflect on angry feelings in a rational and productive manner.

Ingredients:

- 4 drops of blue tansy oil
- 1 drops of wild orange oil
- 100 ml of water
- 2 drops of patchouli oil
- 1 drop of tangerine oil

Instructions: Fill the diffuser container with fresh water (straight from the tap, or distilled or filtered, depending on preference). Add the drops of blue tansy, patchouli, wild orange, and tangerine, then plug in the diffuser and turn it on at the desired setting.

SERENITY NOW

Are you seeing red? Before you do anything you might later regret, take a moment to diffuse this blend. The bergamot, sandalwood, and chamomile are the perfect aromas to help restore or keep your inner cool.

Ingredients:

★ 4 drops of bergamot oil

★ 2 drops of sandalwood oil

★ 2 drops of chamomile oil

★ IOO ml of water

Instructions: Fill the diffuser container with fresh water (straight from the tap, or distilled or filtered, depending on preference). Add the drops of bergamot, sandalwood, and chamomile, then plug in the diffuser and turn it on at the desired setting.

For additional consideration: This blend is particularly effective to calm heightened emotions and soothe the pain of angry of hurt feelings. After several deep breaths, you should find your nerves calmer and your mind ready to consider matters with serenity and wisdom.

RELEASE

The grapefruit, bergamot, and geranium in this blend are wonderful aromas to help release negative forces in both the body and spirit. Whether you need to rid yourself of emotional baggage or muscular tension, this blend is a great, natural way to let it go.

Ingredients:

★ 4 drops of grapefruit oil
★ 3 drops of bergamot oil
★ I drop of geranium oil
★ IOO ml of water

Instructions: Fill the diffuser container with fresh water (straight from the tap, or distilled or filtered, depending on preference). Add the drops of grapefruit, bergamot, and geranium, then plug in the diffuser and turn it on at the desired setting.

For additional consideration: Take in several deep inhales of this aromatic bouquet, and with every exhale visualize yourself releasing tension, negativity, and anything else holding you back. In a few breaths you'll be feeling lighter of spirit and ready to move forward with positivity and strength.

DON'T WORRY, BE HAPPY

My favorite great uncle used to love to sing-song *Don't worry, be happy!* in times of strife. For some reason, it always worked to cheer everyone up. That beloved relative is sadly no longer on this earth but luckily I've found that this blend of rose, lavender, mandarin, and vetiver oils produces a very similar effect to his cheerful singsong of *Don't worry, be happy!*

Ingredients:

★ 3 drops of mandarin oil

★ 2 drops of lavender oil

★ 100 ml of water

★ 2 drops of rose oil

★ 1 drop of vetiver oil

Instructions: Fill the diffuser container with fresh water (straight from the tap, or distilled or filtered, depending on preference). Add the drops of mandarin, rose, lavender, and vetiver, then plug in the diffuser and turn it on at the desired setting.

For additional consideration: A few breaths of this light, floral blend will help reduce anxiety and promote happiness. It may not be quite the same as a dearly beloved relative cheering you up in person but it sure is a close second!

CHEER UP

Here's another wonderful blend that offers a true pick me up when you're feeling low. It even acts as an effective supplement for people looking to treat depression. The valerian root oil in this mix really packs an uplifting punch, so go ahead and prepare this diffusion to get yourself cheered up fast...the natural way!

Ingredients:

★ 4 drops of frankincense oil

★ 1 drop of rosemary oil

★ 100 ml of water

★ 2 drops of lemongrass oil

★ 1 drop of valerian root oil

Instructions: Fill the diffuser container with fresh water (straight from the tap, or distilled or filtered, depending on preference). Add the drops of frankincense, lemongrass, rosemary, and valerian root, then plug in the diffuser and turn it on at the desired setting.

For additional consideration: With a few breaths of this diffusion, your spirits will lift and you will find yourself seeing all the positives around you. Inhale deeply and smile. Have a wonderful day!

HAPPY PLACE

This fun and vibrant blend of patchouli, orange, and lavender is wonderful to lift your mood and stimulate an atmosphere of relaxation and happiness. This is a great combination of aromas to diffuse if you're having a party, or if you're home alone and just want to feel like you're having a party!

Ingredients:

★ 4 drops of patchouli oil
★ 2 drops of orange oil
★ I drop of lavender oil
★ IOO ml of water

Instructions: Fill the diffuser container with fresh water (straight from the tap, or distilled or filtered, depending on preference). Add the drops of patchouli, orange, and lavender, then plug in the diffuser and turn it on at the desired setting.

For additional consideration: This vibrant and uplifting blend will invoke joy and laughter in any space, so breathe deeply, find a smile creeping onto your face, and let the fun begin!

PARTY TIME

Got a party going on and want to make sure that the atmosphere is truly festive? Take a minute to diffuse this good time blend of clary sage, ylang-ylang, peppermint, and sandalwood. These invigorating and stimulating oils will help create a party atmosphere and make your event one to remember.

Ingredients:

★ 4 drops of clary sage oil   ★ 2 drops of ylang-ylang oil

★ 2 drops of peppermint oil   ★ I drop of sandalwood oil

★ IOO ml of water

Instructions: Fill the diffuser container with fresh water (straight from the tap, or distilled or filtered, depending on preference). Add the drops of clary sage, ylang-ylang, peppermint, and sandalwood, then plug in the diffuser and turn it on at the desired setting.

For additional consideration: This fun and lively blend is the perfect way to enhance the atmosphere at any party. A few deep breaths and everyone in the room will feel themselves in the mood to kick the fun up a notch, so inhale deeply and have a great time!

HEALING FORGIVENESS

Showing magnanimity to those who have wronged us can have a powerful effect on our own contentment and happiness. For those times when forgiveness needs a little help, this blend combines the powerful extract of ylang-ylang, known to dispel negative feelings, with the goodwill inducing aromas of soothing sandalwood and grounding vetiver.

Ingredients:

★ 4 drops of ylang-ylang oil
★ 2 drops of sandalwood oil
★ 2 drops of vetiver oil
★ 100 ml of water

Instructions: Fill the diffuser container with fresh water (straight from the tap, or distilled or filtered, depending on preference). Add the drops of ylang-ylang, sandalwood, and vetiver, then plug in the diffuser and turn it on at the desired setting.

For additional consideration: This is a great recipe to use when you need to summon your most generous self. Before confronting those who need to ask your forgiveness, spend several minutes breathing in these aromas and finding your empathetic center.

FAMILY BONDING

Familial relationships are sacred and deserve to be treated that way. Try this aromatic blend in your diffuser next time you're spending quality time with your loved ones. The lemon in this mix is not only refreshing and cleansing, it also helps stimulate natural oxytocin production in the brain, which in turn generates feelings of love and closeness. The lavender and rosemary in this blend balance the lemon perfectly, enhancing sensations of goodwill and affection.

Ingredients:

★ 3 drops of lemon oil

★ 3 drops of lavender oil

★ 3 drops of rosemary oil

★ 100 ml of water

Instructions: Fill the diffuser container with fresh water (straight from the tap, or distilled or filtered, depending on preference). Add the drops of lemon, rosemary, and lavender, then plug in the diffuser and turn it on at the desired setting.

For additional consideration: This is a wonderful recipe to use during family mealtimes, or whenever the family is spending time together and you want to foster feelings of closeness. The blend is gentle enough to use in the evenings, though perhaps not right before bedtime when children are in the space.

SPIRITUAL JOURNEY

This blend can be useful to anyone (religious, non religious, or in between) as they seek to deepen their spiritual connection with the divine. The myrrh has a deeply enlightening effect, opening our minds up to wisdom within and beyond; while the sandalwood is balancing and quieting, allowing us to be maximally attuned to insights and revelations.

Ingredients:

★ 3 drops of myrrh oil
★ 3 drops of sandalwood oil
★ 100 ml of water

Instructions: Fill the diffuser container with fresh water (straight from the tap, or distilled or filtered, depending on preference). Add the drops of myrrh and sandalwood, then plug in the diffuser and turn it on at the desired setting.

For additional consideration: This recipe is best saved for moments of personal or communal holiness. It's an excellent blend to have in the diffuser during church, temple services, or simply to have in the home during prayer or on days of Sabbath. Breathe deeply, and whatever your faith...know that the divine exists in all of us.

SPIRIT SCENTS

Here's another wonderful blend that is perfect to help heighten your being and put you in touch with all that is divine in the world...and in yourself. Use this blend any time you want to tap into a higher power, whatever it may be.

Ingredients:

★ 2 drops of sandalwood oil
★ 2 drops of cedarwood oil
★ 2 drops of lavender oil
★ 2 drops of frankincense oil
★ 2 drops of myrrh oil
★ 100 ml of water

Instructions: Fill the diffuser container with fresh water (straight from the tap, or distilled or filtered, depending on preference). Add the drops of sandalwood, cedarwood, lavender, frankincense, and myrrh, then plug in the diffuser and turn it on at the desired setting.

For additional consideration: This diffusion will delight and nourish your soul. After just a few deep breaths, you'll find yourself in the perfect mood to pray, meditate, or simply reflect on all the wonders of the universe.

TRUE ROMANCE

A perfect blend to user with your sweetheart, this recipe mixes the rich, woodsy aroma of sandalwood oil with the exotic and stimulating jasmine extract. A touch of cypress adds the thrill of the wild to this sultry sweet recipe, setting the ideal mood for an intimate and special time.

Ingredients:

★ 3 drops of sandalwood oil

★ 3 drops of jasmine oil

★ 2 drops of cypress oil

★ 100 ml of water

Instructions: Fill the diffuser container with fresh water (straight from the tap, or distilled or filtered, depending on preference). Add the drops of sandalwood, jasmine, and cypress, then plug in the diffuser and turn it on at the desired setting.

For additional consideration: This cool mist blend will heighten and arouse all the senses, meaning even a simple hug or kiss will feel wonderfully intense. Enjoy being together and take a few deep breaths before the truly heavy breathing begins!

SUPER SATISFACTION

Who said they can't get no satisfaction? It's more attainable than ever with this wonderful blend, which uses cypress to stimulate a deep sense of contentment with the uplifting essences of tangerine and lime. This non-floral blend is an excellent choice for the workplace or any other public setting, as well as the home — really, anywhere that people might want an excuse to pause, breathe deeply, and feel grateful to be alive.

Ingredients:

- ★ 4 drops of cypress oil
- ★ 2 drops of lime oil
- ★ 2 drops of tangerine oil
- ★ 100 ml of water

Instructions: Fill the diffuser container with fresh water (straight from the tap, or distilled or filtered, depending on preference). Add the drops of cypress, tangerine, and lime, then plug in the diffuser and turn it on at the desired setting.

For additional consideration: There is no bad time of day or night to enjoy this recipe, which is perfectly balanced between calming and energizing. With a few breaths, your emotions and awareness will be uplifted and refreshed, and your sense of joy in the world will be shining bright.

48082184R00129

Made in the USA
San Bernardino, CA
15 April 2017